fit for life

BREATHE
EASIER

Credits:

Art Director: Peter Bridgewater
Editorial Consultants: Maria Pal/Clark Robinson Ltd

Picture credits:

key: a = above; b = below

The author and publishers have made every effort to identify the
copyright owners of the photographs; they apologize for any
omissions and wish to thank the following:

David Burch, 73, 89; Mary Evans, 79a; Paul Forrester, 8, 9;
Richard and Sally Greenhill, 77; John Heseltine, 36; Keystone
Press, 79b; Nicholas Laboratories, 10; Science Photo Library, 60;
Chris Thomson, 49, 50, 51, 68, 92, 95; John Watney, 34, 40, 41,
54, 69; Trevor Wood, 55.

fit for life

BREATHE EASIER

VIRGINIA HOPKINS AND ANN PETERS

Gallery Books
an imprint of W.H. Smith Publishers, Inc.
112 Madison Avenue, New York
New York 10016

A QUARTO BOOK

This edition published in 1990 by Gallery Books,
an imprint of W.H. Smith Publishers, Inc.,
112, Madison Avenue, New York, New York 10016

Gallery Books are available for bulk purchase for
sales promotions and premium use. For details write or
telephone the Manager of Special Sales, W.H. Smith
Publishers Inc., 112 Madison Avenue, New York, New
York 10016. (212) 532-6600.

ISBN 0-8317-3897-9

The information and recommendations contained in this book
are intended to complement, not substitute for, the advice of
your own physician. Before starting any medical treatment,
exercise program or diet, consult your physician. Information is
given without any guarantees on the part of the author and
publisher, and they cannot be held responsible for the contents
of this book.

▶ CONTENTS

THE SHOULDERS

Our shoulders are like coat hangers — our bodes hang from them. We often store chronic, stress-related tension in the muscles of the shoulders. We "take the weight of the world on our shoulders;" we "shoulder burdens" and give people the "cold shoulder." Stress-related tension in the shoulders can in turn cause headaches, and can throw out the muscles in the back and hips.

Our muscles work by contracting — in fact, they only contract, or exert a pull. Muscles are connected at each end to bones; when they contract, it's as if the muscle is trying to pull the ends of the bone together. It is this simple movement that allows a weightlifter to heave enormous barbells onto his shoulders, yet also allows a piano player to tickle the ivories.

The trapezius muscles in the shoulders give us an enormous range of movement in our arms, shoulders, and spine, but since they are also the body's "hanger," they work hard most of the time. Physically, muscular tension in the upper shoulders is caused when a contracted muscle fails to relax all the way. This happens frequently in most of the muscles in the body, but the shoulders tend to get more abuse. We do things like hold the phone between our ear and our shoulder and then fail to let the shoulder relax back into its original position. We get depressed and slouch, and the

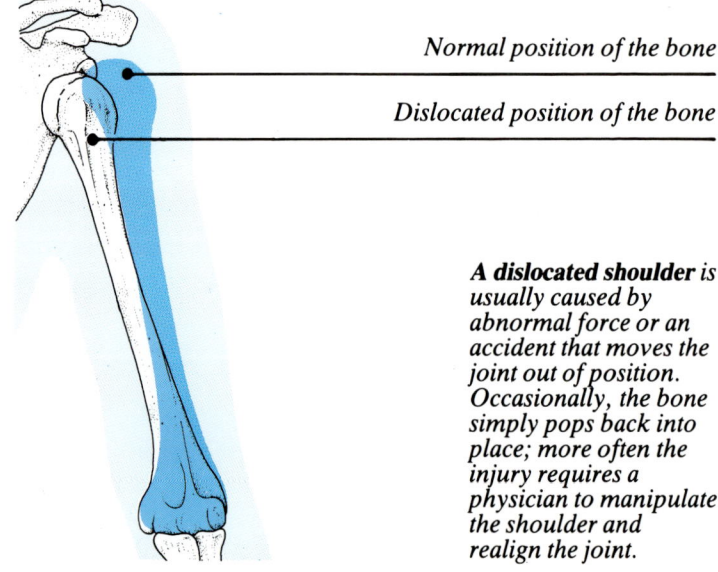

Normal position of the bone

Dislocated position of the bone

A dislocated shoulder is usually caused by abnormal force or an accident that moves the joint out of position. Occasionally, the bone simply pops back into place; more often the injury requires a physician to manipulate the shoulder and realign the joint.

shoulders drop forward. Or we get tense and hold our shoulders unnaturally high.

One of the best and most pleasant treatments for tense, sore, and overcontracted shoulder muscles is a shoulder massage. Warmth, from a heating pad or even the sun, will help. Relaxation techniques such as deep-breathing and meditation can help release the shoulder muscles. There are also exercise routines that involve contracting and relaxing the shoulder muscles; these can be very helpful as long as the exercise leaves the muscles in an uncontracted state.

One of the most common shoulder injuries is dislocating the shoulder. The muscles that extend from the shoulder over the upper arm hold the arms in place and allow wide rotation of the arm joint. Sometimes the muscle fibers are so stretched during a sudden or violent movement, that the upper arm bone pulls out of position and "dislocates." Sometimes the bone will pop right back into place; often it must be manipulated back into position. In either case, a doctor should be consulted quickly.

MUSCLES THAT MOVE THE UPPER SHOULDER

The trapezius muscle holds the shoulder blade in position and rotates it. This muscle also draws the head back and to the side.

The deltoid muscle covers the shoulder joint. It raises and rotates the arm.

The triceps muscle joins the shoulder to the elbow and contracts to extend the forearm.

The pectoralis major is the large shoulder muscle that lies across the chest. It can draw the arm forward and rotate it.

The sternomastoid inclines the head towards the shoulder of the same side or rotates it towards the other side.

The biceps brachii muscle runs from the shoulder to the ulna in the forearm.

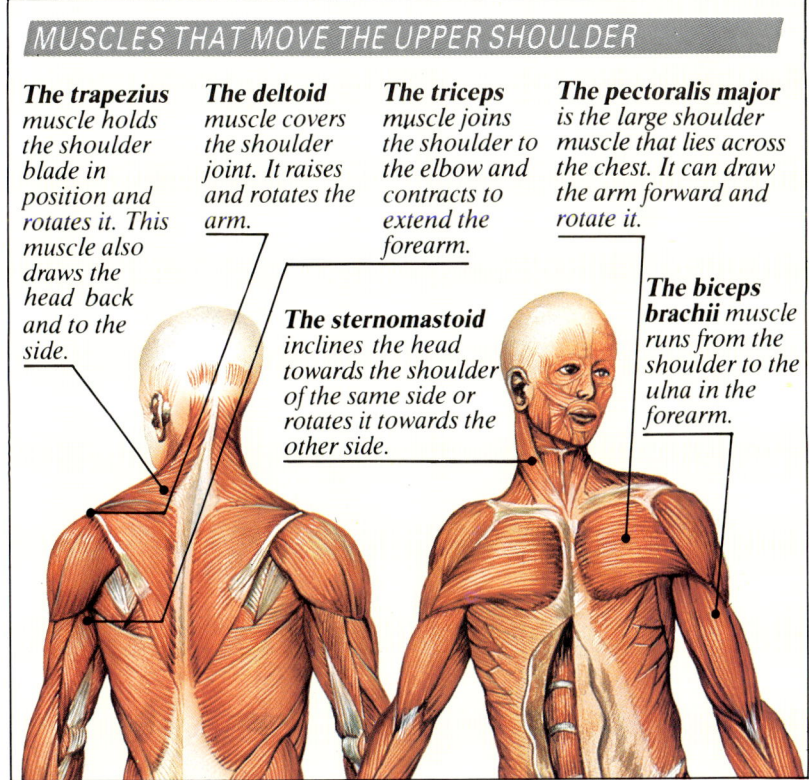

▶ HEAD AND SHOULDERS WARM-UPS

Too many of us ignore exercising the head, neck and shoulder areas. Since most sports require quick responses and eye–hand coordination, many times a snap of the head results in a pulled muscle. So if you really want to be able to put your nose to the grindstone and excel at your sport, let's warm up the head and shoulders!

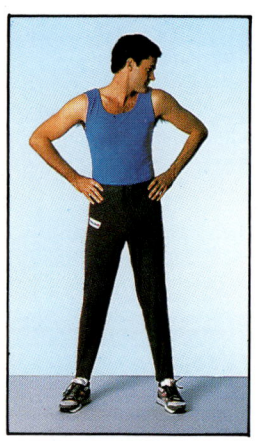
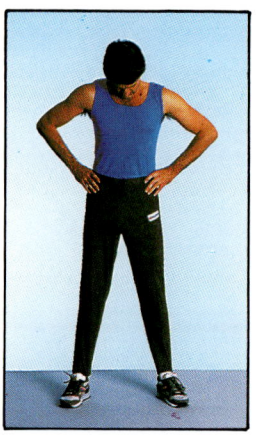
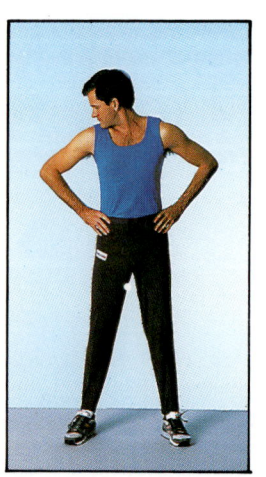
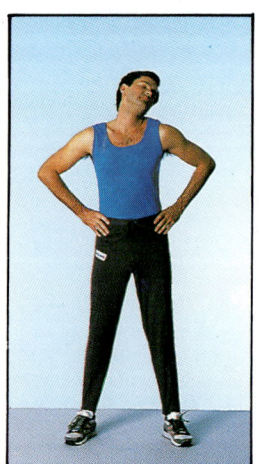

HEAD ROLLS

Stand erect, keep feet apart with hands on hips and place chin on left shoulder.

Slowly drop chin until it touches chest.

Then roll the chin up to the right shoulder.

Then tilt chin up as you roll your head until the chin rests again on the left shoulder. Repeat in a continuous motion 10 times (10×).

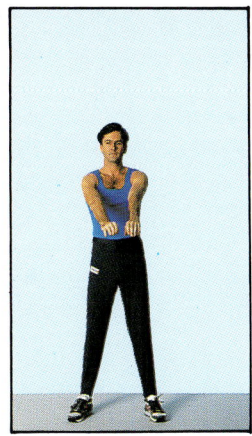 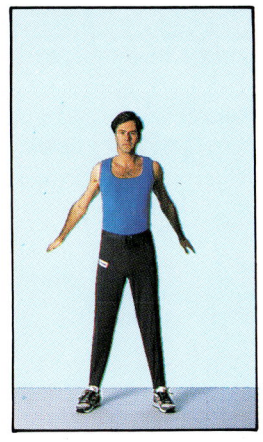 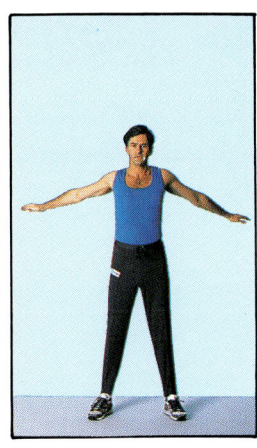

GIANT ARM SWINGS

Stand erect with arms held straight up above the head and drop them slowly in a swinging motion in front of your body.

Continue the motion, bringing your arms past your body.

Complete the movement by swinging arms back up to the starting position. Repeat in a continuous motion 10×.

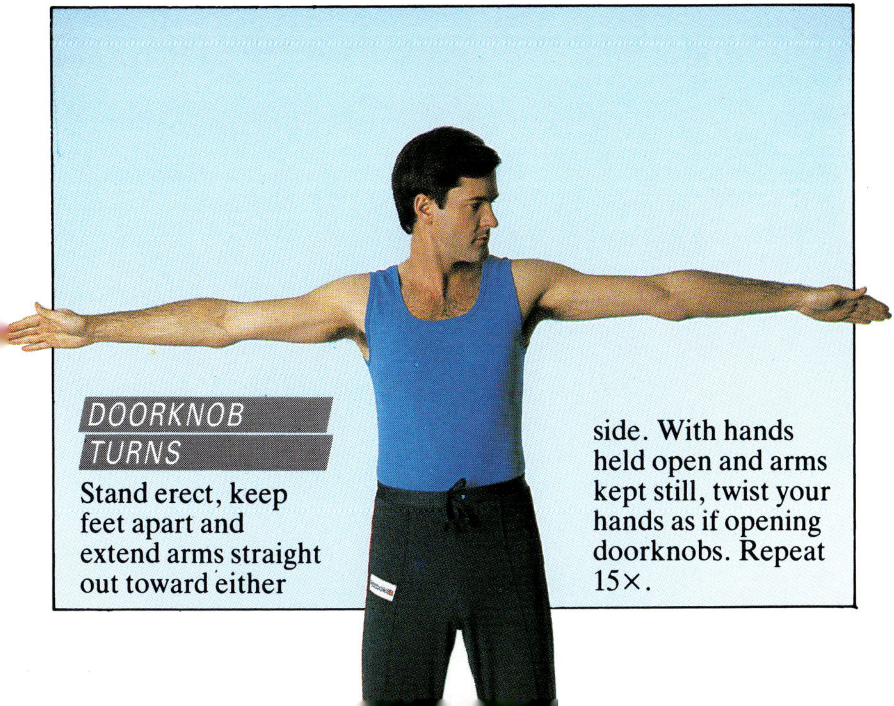

DOORKNOB TURNS

Stand erect, keep feet apart and extend arms straight out toward either side. With hands held open and arms kept still, twist your hands as if opening doorknobs. Repeat 15×.

▶ A SIMPLE SHOULDER MASSAGE

There aren't a lot of things in the world that feel better than a good shoulder massage. People tend to store a lot of tension in the shoulder muscles, so relaxing them can be extremely healing. A shoulder massage is a nice thing to do for friends and family, and can really help when someone is feeling upset, tense, or is in physical pain or discomfort.

Below is a step-by-step description of a wonderfully relaxing and soothing shoulder massage. But first, some suggestions:

🔵 Give a shoulder massage as a gift, when you really want to. If your mind is elsewhere, or if you're not enjoying giving the massage, you may leave your friend feeling worse.

🔵 Focus your mind and your feelings of good will in your hands and fingertips. This will create a sensitivity to the other person, so that the amount of pressure you use is just right.

🔵 The pressure of the hands and fingers should be firm but sensitive. If you come upon a knot in one of the muscles, knead it gently but firmly. If it doesn't melt away fairly quickly, move on to another spot and come back to it later.

🔵 Try to keep at least one hand in contact with the other person's body throughout the massage. This helps maintain a sense of confidence and relaxation in the other person.

🔵 Keep in mind what you would like if you were receiving the massage — human bodies are much more alike than different, and you know what kinds of touch and pressure relieve tension best from personal experience.

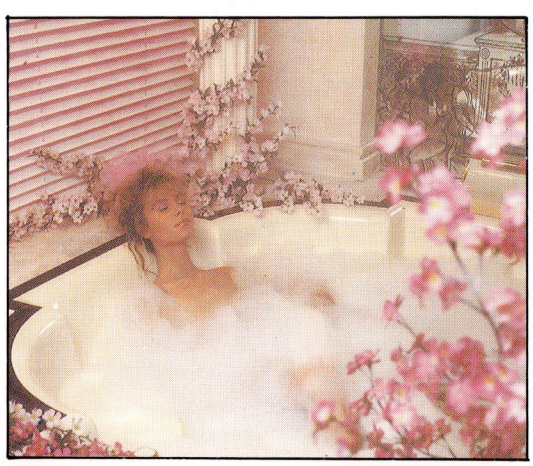

An an alternative to a massage, a hot bath after a hard day's work can be very relaxing and helpful in relieving tension.

MASSAGING THE SHOULDERS

1 Place your palms firmly and gently on the seated person's shoulders. Ask the person to take a few deep breaths with you. This establishes contact and a sense of rapport.

2 Lightly run your hands and/or fingertips up and down the person's shoulders, back, and upper arms.

3 Increase the pressure of your hand some, and rub the back in a quick, circular motion, with the heel of the hand. Cover the entire back, up and down.

4 Now that the person is somewhat relaxed, it's time to move to the shoulders. Grasp the shoulder muscles firmly and slowly knead them. This is the basic shoulder rub. Focus on your fingertips — each one moves separately, and yet they all flow together as well. Knead the muscle smoothly, creating a wave-like flow. Do *not* give the muscles a hard squeeze! Move along the shoulders and down to the upper arms. As you do one arm, put your other hand on the person's other arm or the upper chest as a brace.

5 Drop the thumbs down to between the shoulder blades and knead the muscles there as well. Avoid digging the thumbs in — respond to the give and take of the other person's muscles.

6 Work along the tops of the shoulders, back and forth. Lift the large shoulder muscle just below the neck.

7 Using the thumbs, press firmly down on points along the shoulder, beginning at the outside of the shoulder and working in. If there is tenderness in the shoulder muscles, be gentle. It is often effective to have the other person take a deep breath; as he or she exhales, press slowly into the point. As the person inhales again, release the pressure slowly, and so on.

8 Now move to the neck area. Place one hand on the person's forehead to brace the head, and with the other gently "pinch" the muscles that run on either side of the spine from the shoulders to the base of the skull.

9 Use your thumb and forefinger to make small circles along the base of the skull. Then, using the thumb, press in and up at the depression just under the base of the skull. Now work the points along the base of the skull with the thumb; follow the same breathing techniques as in step 7 above.

10 Gently and briskly rub the sides and top of the person's head with your fingers, working gradually toward the shoulders again. When you get to their shoulders, make gentle "chopping" motions along the shoulders and down the back. Avoid the spine and work very gently around the kidney area under the ribs.

11 Lightly run your hands along the shoulders and back as in step 1.

▶ *THE NECK*

The neck is one of the most beautiful, graceful, useful, and important parts of the human body. It is the support structure for the head, which on most adults weighs an average of 15 to 20 pounds — yet the head rotates easily and effortlessly. The neck is also the main passageway between the brain and the rest of the body. It is a crossroads for all sensory and bodily information going to and from the brain, and it houses the cervical vertebrae of the spinal column.

The neck is an extremely strong, yet supple, structure. It has a wider range and more variety of movement available to it than any other joint in the body. Although most joints have only two bones, there are seven bones in the neck joint. These bones are called the cervical vertebrae (*cervical* meaning neck). Because the neck is such a complex structure, and is vulnerable to forces from every direction, it is also susceptible to a lot of complications.

The seven vertebrae of the neck are part of the spine. The unusual shape of the vertebrae allows the muscles of the neck to attach to the spine at many different angles.

The first or uppermost vertebra is called the atlas, and this is where the weight of the head is supported. Most people think their neck ends at about the bottom of the ear lobes. But if you feel the back of your head at the base of the skull, you'll get a sense of how long your neck really is.

The second bone of the neck vertebrae is called the axis. The head pivots on this bone with support from the other five cervical vertebrae, much the way a globe rotates on its axis. However, thanks to the flexibility of the five remaining vertebrae, your head has a much greater range of motion than a globe does. The head can move forward and backward, up and down, and side to side, as well as in a circular motion. The nerves that radiate through the cervical vertebrae include those that regulate the muscles of the eyes, the mouth, the lungs, and the heart.

The framework of the neck can be disrupted by injury, by chronic misuse such as poor posture, and by short-term misuse or injury, such as straining the neck for some reason.

WHIPLASH

Whiplash is a common neck injury that is often the result of being in a car that is rear-ended by another car. The head is thrown forward violently by the force of the blow and then "whipped" back suddenly. When the head is thrown forward suddenly in a whiplash

THE NECK AND POSTURE

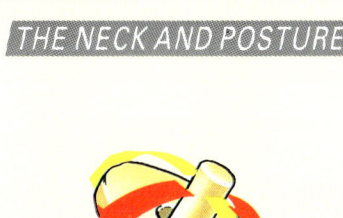

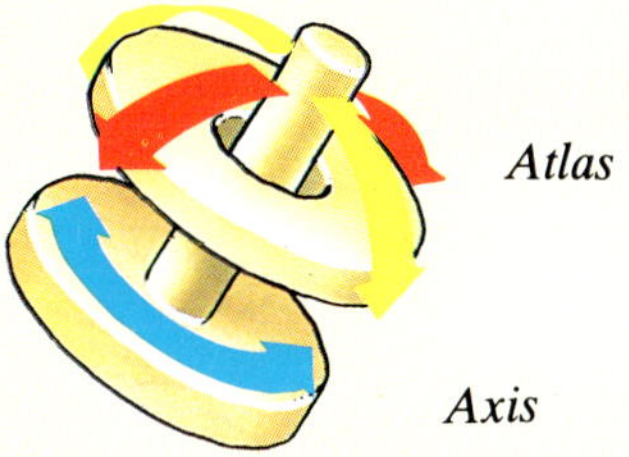

Atlas

Axis

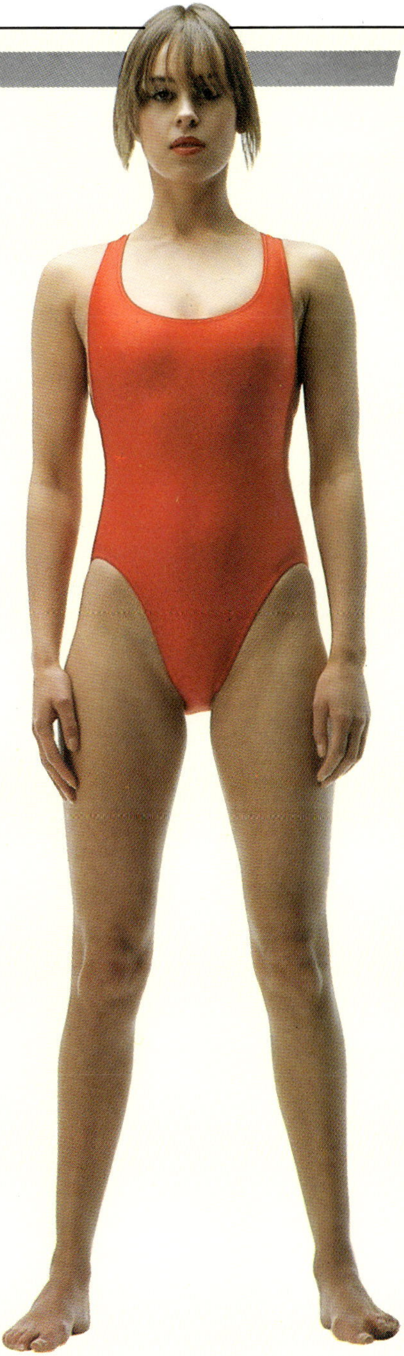

The wide range of *movements we can make with our head, rotating it, nodding up and down, are made possible by a pivot joint (above) situated between the first two vertebrae of the neck — the atlas and axis.*

Persistent poor posture *is a common cause of neck ache and injury. When standing for long periods it is particularly easy to fall into bad habits, such as slouching and letting the head fall forward, putting strain on the neck. Try to keep the head level and your chin up (right); the shoulders and back should be straight but relaxed. Rather than shifting from one foot to another, distribute your weight evenly on both feet, which will help reduce fatigue and stress to other body parts.*

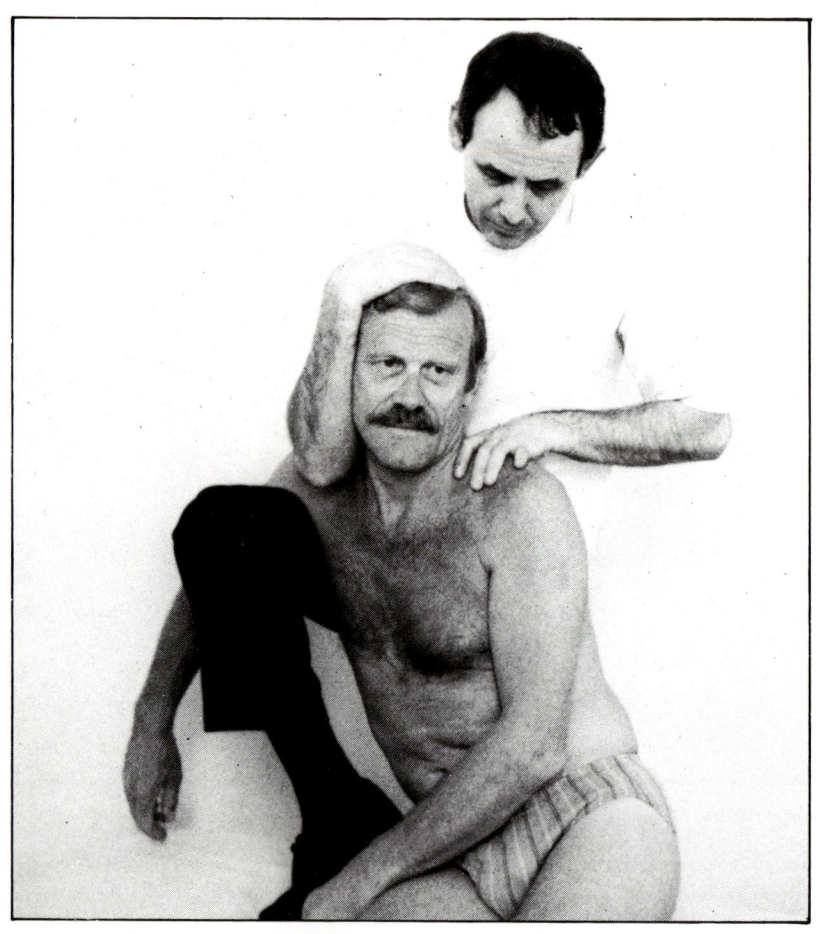

Osteopathic manipulation *for joints at the nape of the neck.*

accident, the muscles of the neck are pulled violently, then contracted violently. This often pulls or pushes the cervical vertebrae out of alignment. The frequency and severity of whiplash injuries to front-seat passengers have gone down significantly since the use of seat belts and headrests in automobiles — another good reason to wear your seat belt.

A physician should be consulted for any serious neck injury, including whiplash. X rays are often necessary to determine the extent of the injury. Symptoms of whiplash include severe aching in the neck the day after the injury, a limited range of motion of the head, neck muscles locked in painful spasm, and possibly a recurring headache.

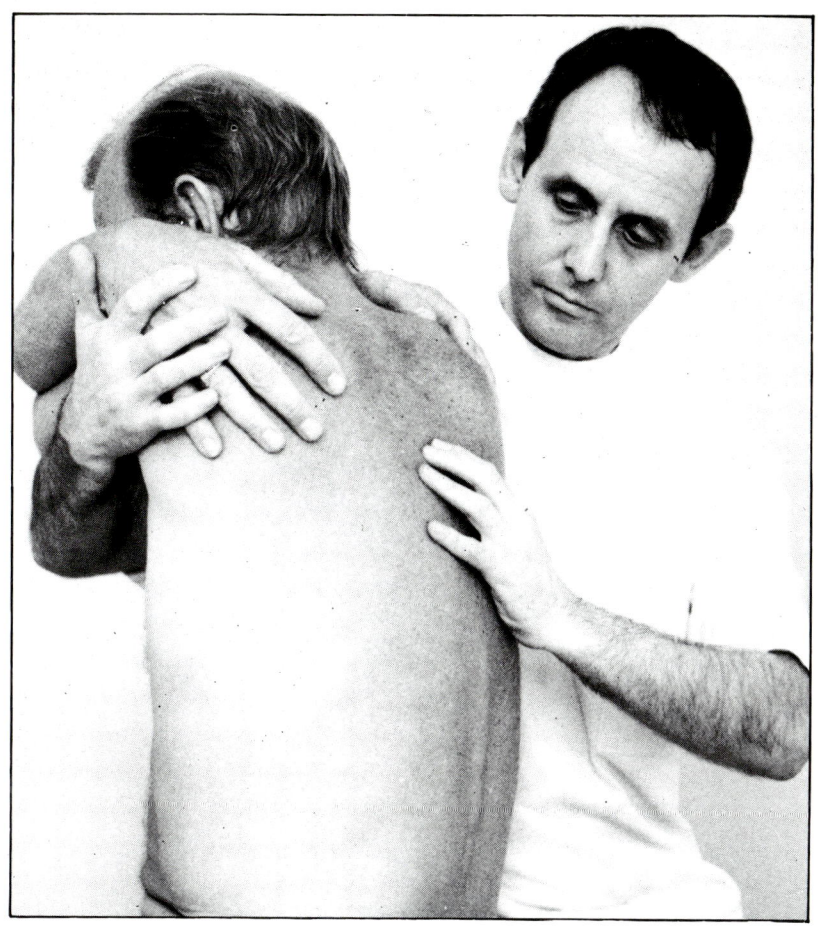

Osteopathic assessment of spinal joints in the thoracic area.

Treatment of whiplash or any neck injury usually includes immobilization of the neck, usually with a neck brace. Hot pads and/or ice packs may be recommended. Physical therapy can sometimes help in the recovery from a whiplash or any other kind of a neck injury. Massage may help to increase the blood circulation to the neck, and in this way assist the body in draining waste products from the injured tissue, and help the muscles loosen from their state of spasm.

Any numbness or paralysis in the face or upper part of the body that occurs as a result of a neck injury is serious and a physician should be consulted immediately. Damage to vital nerves in the neck can have serious consequences.

TAKING CARE OF THE NECK

It is important to give your neck proper support while sleeping. Don't rest your head on too many pillows. Try to turn the whole body with the head, to place less strain on the neck. If the whole spine can move, however subtly, with the neck, the movement is easier and more graceful. Change position frequently when reading or writing so the neck muscles don't become locked in one position. Try to keep cold drafts off the neck while sitting or sleeping, as this often causes the muscles to tense up.

SPINAL MANIPULATION

Spinal manipulation is done by chiropractors, and also osteopathic and naturopathic physicians. It should never be attempted by anyone except a qualified practitioner. It is a process whereby the vertebrae are moved, usually manually, to reposition them back into their correct alignment. Practitioners of spinal manipulation believe that vertebrae which are out of alignment hamper the blood supply and/or affect the nerves between the brain and the rest of the body, eventually causing pain and ill-health in the organs, arms, and legs. During a spinal manipulation there may be a harmless clicking or popping sound caused by the movement of the tendons and ligaments.

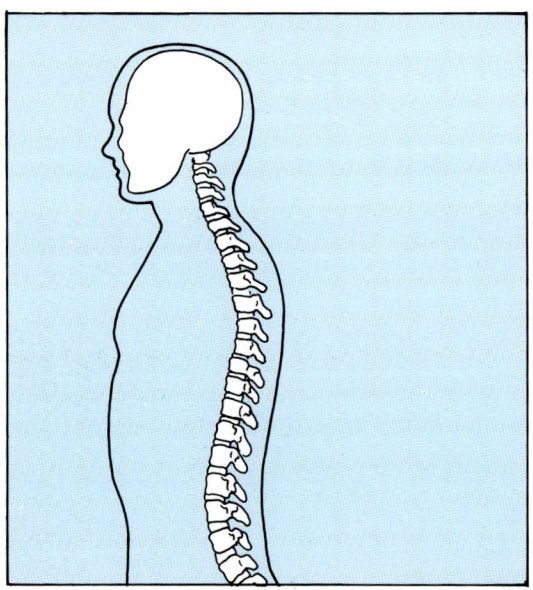

Chiropractors believe that vertebrae out of alignment can influence the health of other organs. Normally, the spine forms a gentle S-shape (left). If this is distorted, a chiropractor aims to reposition the affected vertebrae by spinal manipulation. Part of the diagnosis involves testing the spine for sideways movement (right).

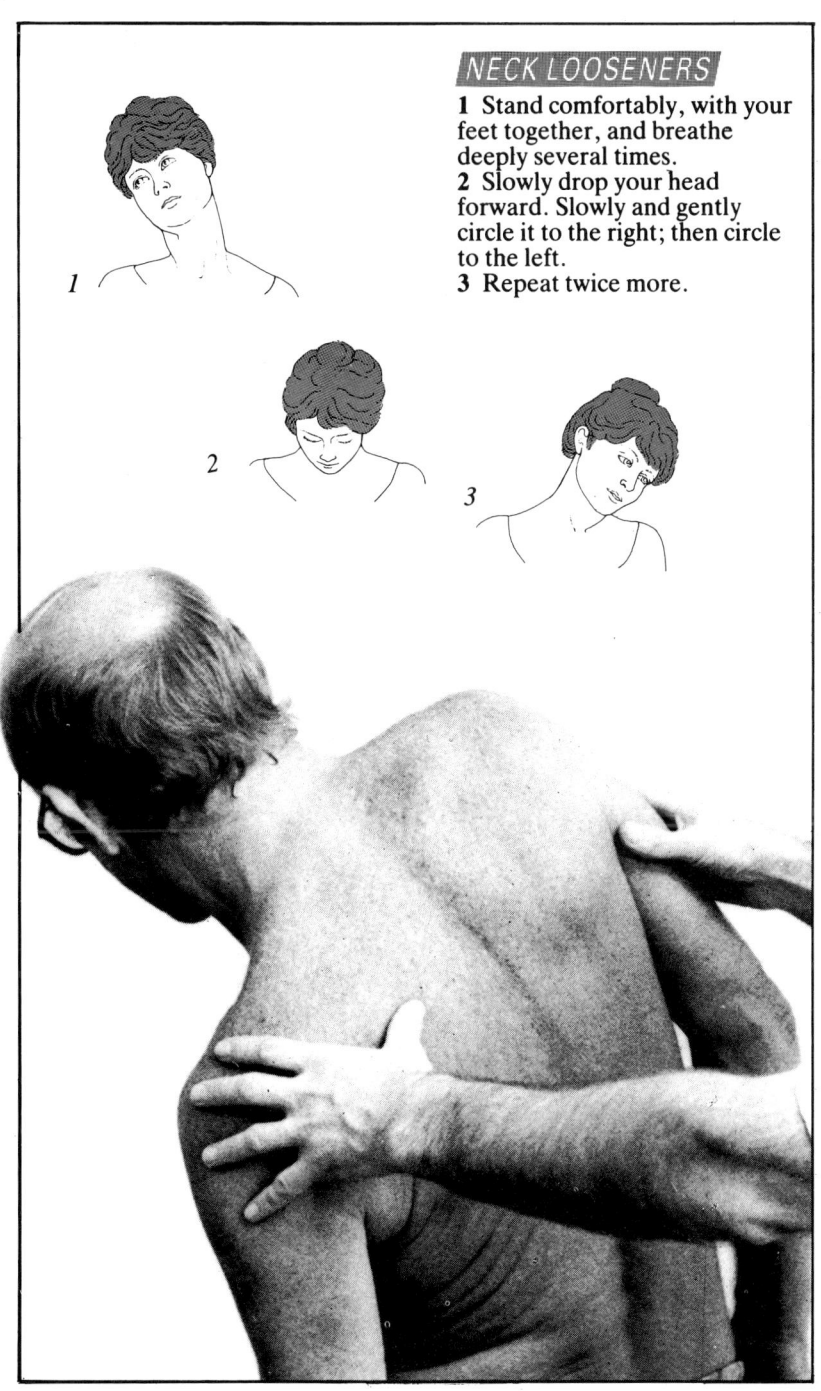

NECK LOOSENERS

1 Stand comfortably, with your feet together, and breathe deeply several times.
2 Slowly drop your head forward. Slowly and gently circle it to the right; then circle to the left.
3 Repeat twice more.

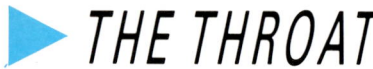

THE THROAT

The throat is the part of the body responsible for passing both air and food from outside the body to the inside, to sustain and nourish it. The trachea or windpipe carries air to and from the lungs, and the esophagus or gullet is a muscular tube that connects the mouth and throat with the stomach.

LARYNGITIS

Laryngitis occurs when the mucous membrane of the larynx (voice box) becomes inflamed. The mucous membrane is a lining that covers and protects the larynx. It's easy to tell when someone has laryngitis, because his or her voice becomes very hoarse or disappears altogether. Other symptoms may include a slight fever and pain or swelling in the region of the larynx. Laryngitis can come on suddenly (acute infection) or occur more gradually (chronic infection).

Laryngitis is caused by a bacterial infection, and often develops during the course of a cold. It can also be caused by other irritations, however, such as atmospheric pollution, smoke, fumes, dust, over-using the voice, or using it incorrectly. Ordinarily there are no dangers directly associated with laryngitis. In rare cases swelling and inflammation may obstruct the air passages in the throat and create difficulty breathing.

The best treatment for laryngitis is resting the voice, to give the inflamed tissues the best conditions to heal themselves. In the winter, humidifying the air with steam may help ease the symptoms. A drink of honey and lemon juice mixed in warm water can help relieve the pain of inflammation. In a severe case of laryngitis a physician may want to prescribe antibiotics. If the condition persists, the larynx should be checked for polyps or tumors.

A general hoarseness in the voice can be caused by anything that prevents the two vocal cords in the throat from meeting normally; the causes may be the same as those for laryngitis. Hoarseness that lasts for more than a few days could indicate a disease of the vocal cords and should be checked by a physician.

Tumors on the larynx are very common, and are usually benign. Some of the symptoms may be hoarseness, coughing, pain, difficulty swallowing, and blood in the saliva. A large tumor may obstruct the airway and create difficulty in breathing. Surgical removal of a tumor or polyp on the larynx can often be a fairly simple office procedure.

THE WINDPIPE

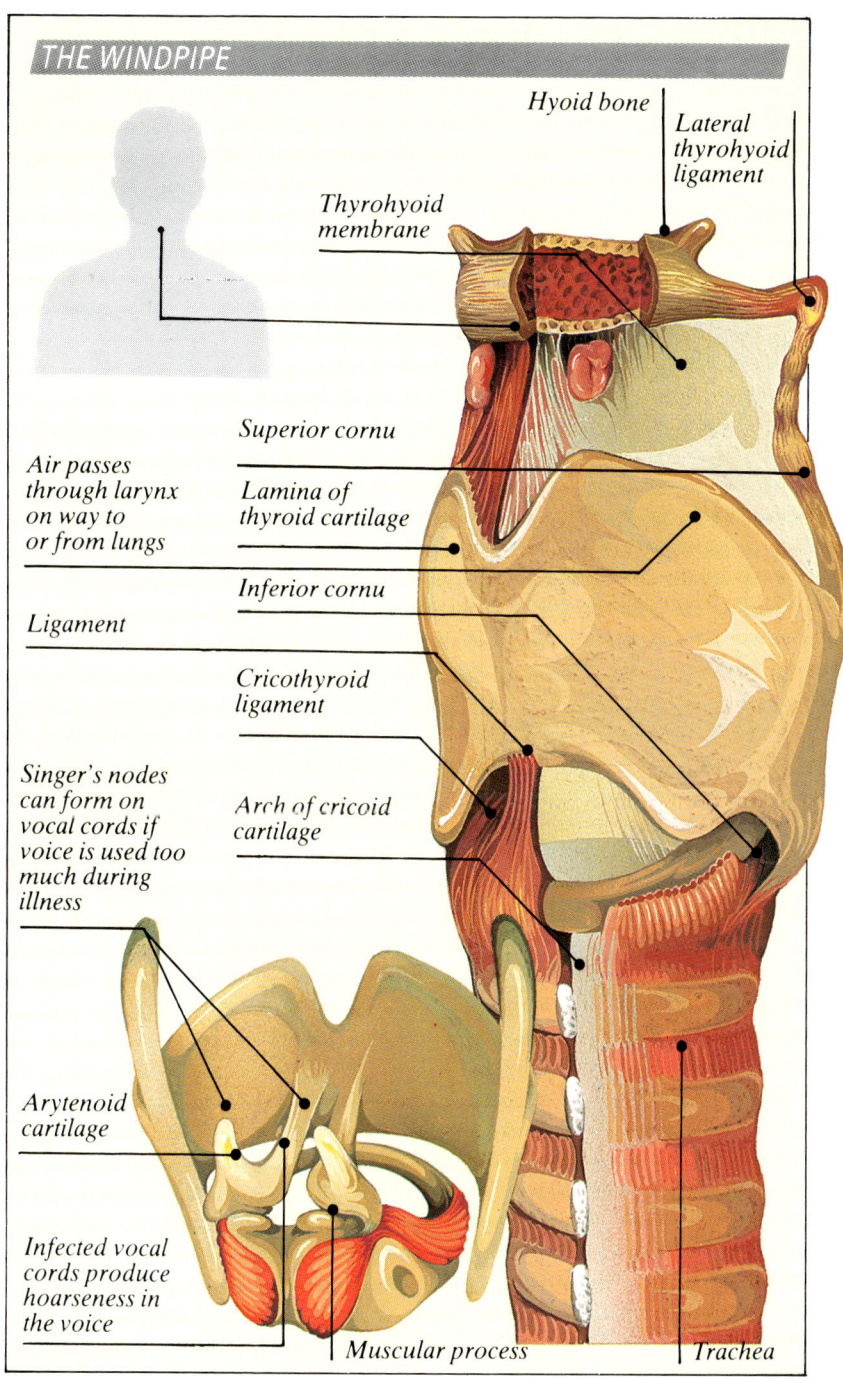

Hyoid bone

Lateral thyrohyoid ligament

Thyrohyoid membrane

Superior cornu

Air passes through larynx on way to or from lungs

Lamina of thyroid cartilage

Inferior cornu

Ligament

Cricothyroid ligament

Singer's nodes can form on vocal cords if voice is used too much during illness

Arch of cricoid cartilage

Arytenoid cartilage

Infected vocal cords produce hoarseness in the voice

Muscular process

Trachea

SORE THROAT

A sore throat is a swelling or inflammation of the lining on the back wall of the throat, and can be caused by an irritant, an infection, or swollen glands. Symptoms of a sore throat include difficulty and pain swallowing, inflammation, and fever. A sore throat sometimes signals the beginning of a cold or flu. A sore throat that doesn't go away can be caused by excess cigarette, pipe or cigar smoking, too much alcohol, a sinus infection, or long-term inhalation of irritating substances.

STREP THROAT

Strep throat, or streptococcus, is a severe form of sore throat. It tends to come on suddenly, and the symptoms include chills and fever, general weakness, and headache. The throat becomes very red and swollen and covered with gray patches. Consult your doctor if you think you have a strep throat.

Antibiotics are not necessarily prescribed for strep throat. Treatment for strep includes plenty of rest, fluids, and a mild, light diet. A mixture of lemon or lime juice, honey, and hot water taken every

TONSILLITIS

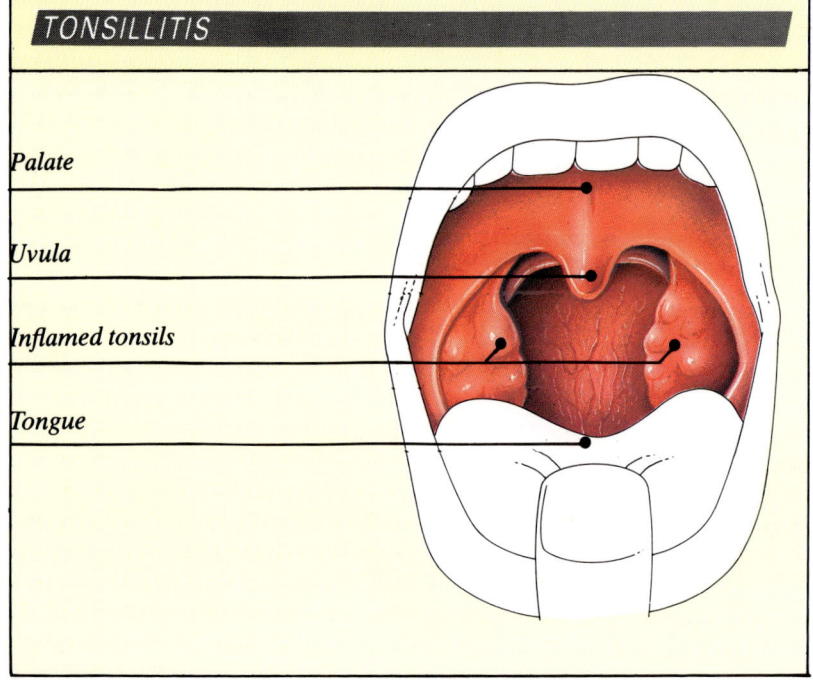

Palate

Uvula

Inflamed tonsils

Tongue

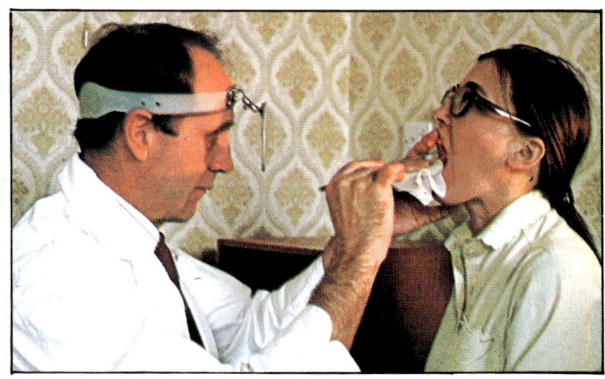

A sore throat *that is accompanied by hoarseness usually indicates an attack of laryngitis, easily confirmed by a throat examination.*

few hours can ease the symptoms. A common home remedy for sore throat is a hot herbal tea made with fresh ginger root, dried sage and dried goldenseal. A gargle of two teaspoons of apple-cider vinegar in a cup of warm water, or a salt water gargle, can also help.

TONSILS

The tonsils are two glandlike structures located above and behind the tongue. When they are healthy, they can barely be seen, but when inflamed they are large, reddened masses with spots of pus on the surface.

The function of the tonsils is to help prevent infections that can enter the body through the nose and the mouth. It used to be that the tonsils were routinely removed surgically from children between the ages of three and five. Nowadays the prevailing wisdom is that the tonsils perform a valuable disease-prevention role in the body and should be removed only when they are no longer functional because of constant infection — tonsillitis.

The symptoms of infected tonsils include pain in the throat area, high fever, swollen glands in the neck, recurrent ear infections and sore throats, and sometimes obstructed breathing.

SWOLLEN GLANDS

Swollen glands are a swelling of the lymph glands located under the jaw or along the side of the neck. The swelling may be caused by infections of the tonsils, a severe sore throat, an infection of the sinuses, swollen adenoids, or mumps. Swollen glands are most often an indication that something else in the body is not functioning properly.

21

THE HEIMLICH MANEUVER

The Heimlich Maneuver is a technique for clearing the air passages when a person is choking on a swallowed object such as a piece of food.

1 First, try gently inserting a finger into the victim's throat to see if the blockage can be removed that way. It's important that this be done carefully so that the blockage isn't pushed farther down the throat.

2 If that isn't successful, grasp the victim from behind and clasp both arms around his or her lower chest. Make a fist with one hand and place if just below the breastbone, under the ribs; and place your other hand over the fist. Give a sudden, sharp, and forceful thrust with the fist inward and upward, by tightening the arms and hands and "hugging" the person. This usually dislodges the foreign object so that it can be coughed up.

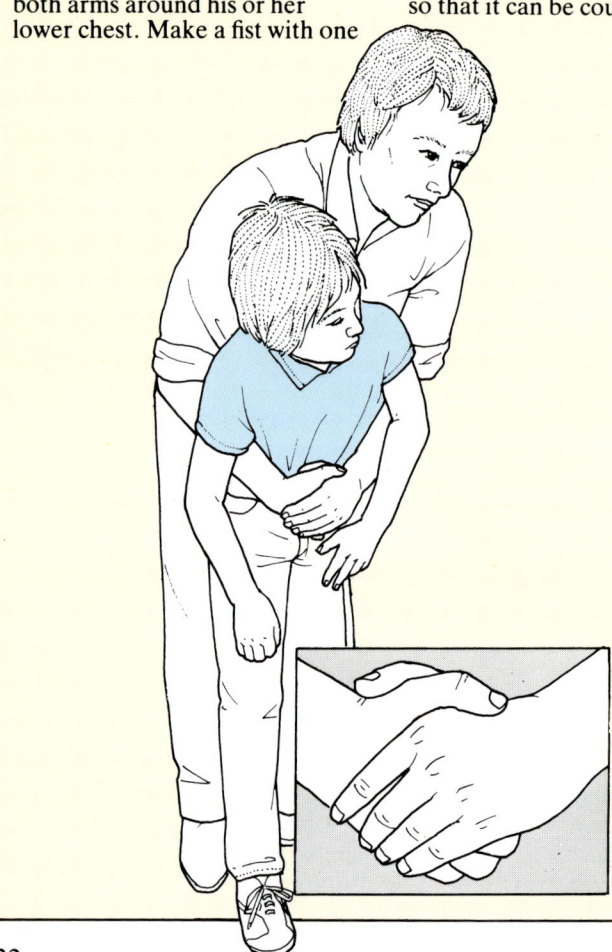

▶ *THE JAWS*

The jaws are the powerful bone and muscle structure around the mouth that holds the teeth and allows us to move our mouth and chew our food.

The jaw can sometimes become infected due to a tooth infection. This condition usually needs to be treated with antibiotics. Sometimes a jaw infection must be surgically drained in order to heal properly. A fractured jaw is a fairly common accident. The symptoms can include pain, swelling, and difficulty chewing. A fractured jaw usually needs to be immobilized by wiring the jaw closed, and can take four to six weeks to heal.

TMJ

TMJ, or temporal-mandibular joint dysfunction, seems to be the stress-related disease of the 1980s. The TMJ (temporal-mandibular joint) is the hinge joint of the jaw, which operates much like the hinge of a door. When one side of a door hinge is loose or off-balance, the other side takes extra wear and tear and the door doesn't close properly. When the "hinge" of the jaw is "off," the muscles that attach the upper and lower parts of the jaw may also be affected. Symptoms of TMJ include headaches, a clamped jaw, clicking in the jaw, and earaches. However, a clicking in the jaw doesn't necessarily indicate TMJ.

One possible cause of TMJ is thought to be improper dental and orthodontic treatment, including supposedly corrective manipulative orthodontic procedures, and poor fitting of dentures, bridges, and fillings. TMJ can also be caused by injury, but it is often caused by emotional stress, which creates nervous habits such as grinding the teeth and rocking and clenching the jaws, which pulls the joint out of line.

The treatment for TMJ can be as simple as learning how to handle stress in more positive ways, thereby reducing the severity of teeth-grinding and clenching and rocking of the jaws. Specially made and fitted bite plates that hold the teeth and jaw in proper alignment are a common TMJ treatment, as is adjusting the bite of the teeth through grinding down or building up the teeth.

Before resorting to expensive dental treatments for TMJ, use a common-sense approach. Look at some of your habits and your lifestyle. Some habits that may cause or aggravate TMJ include holding the telephone receiver between the ear and the shoulder, and chewing gum. Reducing the amount of stress in your life or learning to handle it in different ways can also help.

THE MOUTH

The mouth is our main point of contact with the rest of the world. With our mouths we eat, speak, sing, and generally express ourselves. Since the mouth is a major avenue of expression of the self, any disorder of the mouth, even if not serious, can affect the way we feel about ourselves in general, and in turn affect our health in general.

COLD SORES

A virus called herpes simplex can cause painful blisters and sores to form on the lips and sometimes in the mouth. The infection is often called a cold sore because having a cold can make the virus appear again after an initial attack has gone away. Herpes simplex is very common and there isn't much that can be done about it. A mild case — and most cases are — needs no treatment at all.

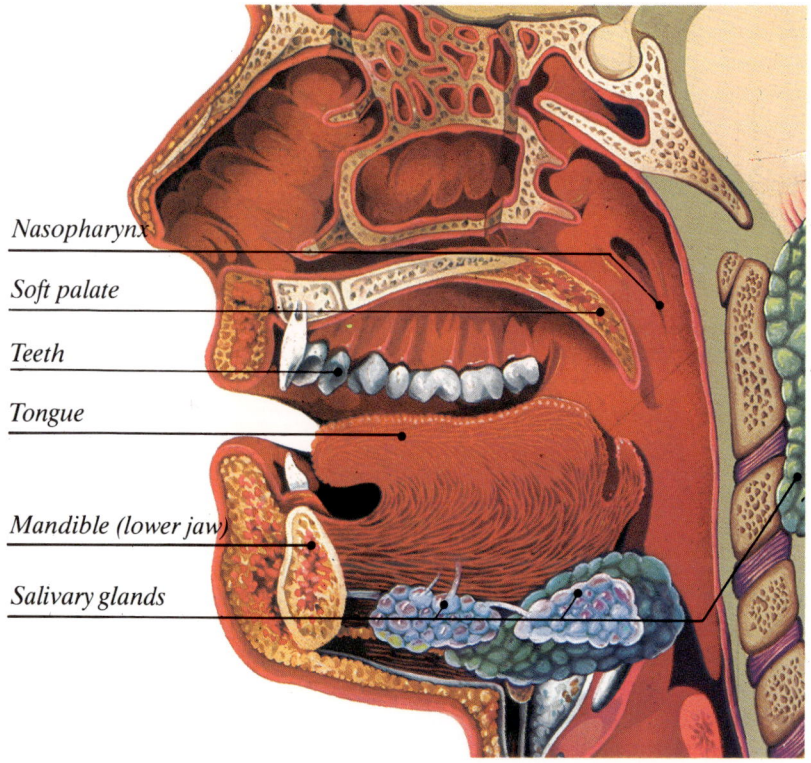

Nasopharynx

Soft palate

Teeth

Tongue

Mandible (lower jaw)

Salivary glands

MOUTH ULCERS

A break in the sensitive lining of the mouth can cause an ulcer — a yellow or white spot with a red rim — to appear. Mouth ulcers can be caused by an injury to the lining, such as biting the inside of your mouth, or being hit in the mouth by something. A broken tooth or badly fitting denture can also cause a mouth ulcer. Canker sores are a type of mouth ulcer that can often appear in people who are under stress, or ill, or run down in general. Most mouth ulcers simply go away by themselves in a few days. However, if the ulcer is caused by a dental problem, see your dentist. See your doctor if any other mouth ulcers don't heal within ten days or so, or if they recur often. Nonprescription gels and liquids that numb the area help relieve the pain. Avoid eating spicy or acidic foods while the ulcer is painful.

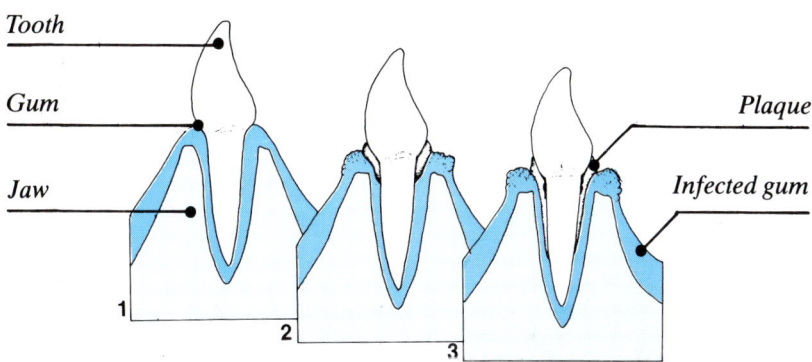

Tooth

Gum

Jaw

Plaque

Infected gum

1

2

3

Many people suffer *to some degree from gingivitis — inflammation of the gums — and may experience slight bleeding when they brush their teeth. It is caused by plaque that* *accumulates between the teeth and the gums. Bacterial poisons from the plaque create tiny ulcers at the edges of the gums which consequently become infected and swollen.*

GINGIVITIS

Swollen and inflamed gums can indicate gingivitis, a very common dental problem in adults. Plaque, the sticky deposit of food particles and bacteria that forms on teeth, is thought to irritate the gums and make them become inflamed. If you have gingivitis, your gums are red and soft and bleed easily.

The best treatment for gingivitis is prevention and the best prevention is to follow the rules of good dental hygiene. Brush your teeth after every meal and use dental floss regularly. See your dentist at least once a year for a check-up. If gingivitis is untreated, it can lead to more serious gum disease and possible loss of teeth.

BAD BREATH

Bad breath, or halitosis, is usually a temporary condition that can be caused by a wide variety of factors. One of the most common causes of bad breath is simply eating foods such as garlic or onions that leave an odor on the breath, or getting food particles such as meat caught between the teeth, which then decay and create an odor. Smoking, certain medications, alcohol and a variety of diseases of the lungs, stomach, liver and kidneys can also cause bad breath. Poor digestion can cause "fumes" that rise from the stomach.

Diseases in the mouth such as infections of the tongue, jaws, teeth, and gums can create bad breath.

The treatment of bad breath begins with good health and proper oral hygiene, including brushing and flossing the teeth regularly. A dentist of physician should be consulted when bad breath is persistant, as it may be an indication of infection or disease.

THE TONGUE

The tongue is our organ of taste and an important organ of speech. It has also been used by physicians for centuries to help diagnose disease. The color, shape, and texture of the tongue can be a general indicator of health. The tongue also transmits information about taste to the brain. The tongue may get red and irritated from being burned by hot or spicy food, tobacco, and alcohol. Rough teeth, improperly fitted dentures, vitamin deficiencies, and allergic reactions can also cause tongue irritations.

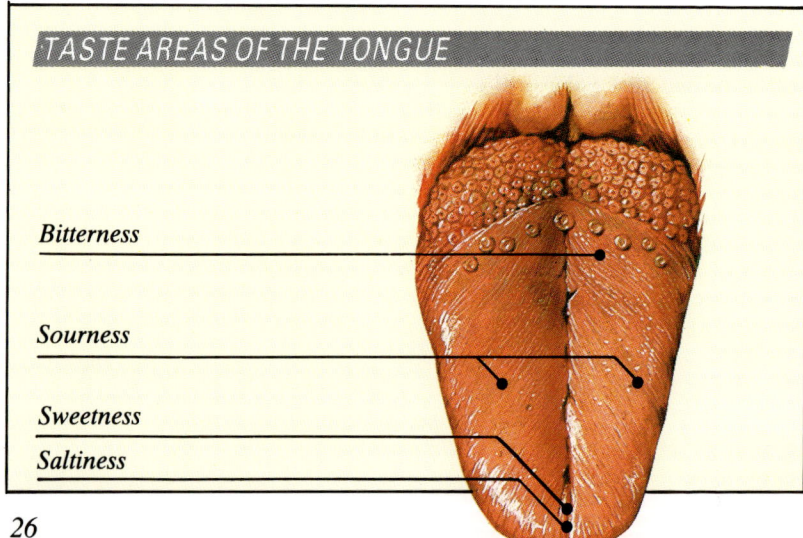

TASTE AREAS OF THE TONGUE

Bitterness

Sourness

Sweetness

Saltiness

THE TEETH

We have two sets of teeth in our lifetimes — baby and adult. Baby teeth begin to grow in at about six months of age and continue to come in until about the age of two. Then around the age of six the baby teeth begin falling out, to be replaced by adult teeth, which are usually completely grown in by the age of 12.

Proper dental hygiene is by far the most important factor for most people in maintaining healthy teeth. Cavities are formed when food is not cleaned from the teeth after eating. Carbohydrates and sugars left on the teeth are transformed into acids by the bacteria normally present in the mouth. The acid breaks down the protective enamel of the teeth, eventually creating a cavity. Cavities can create serious toothaches and abscesses or infections, if they are not treated by professional dentistry. The symptoms of an abscess are swelling, pain, and redness in the area of the tooth. A dentist often needs to prescribe antibiotics to treat an abscessed tooth.

Good oral and dental hygiene includes regular brushing and flossing of the teeth and gums, and annual visits to the dentist for cleaning and to check for cavities and other problems. Your toothbrush should have close-set, straight-topped bristles that don't irritate your gums — in order to prevent it becoming worn and developing uneven, damaging surfaces, be sure to replace it often. Brushing should be in a circular downward motion on the top teeth and gums, and in a circular upward motion on the bottom teeth. It's important to reach back and brush the back teeth well, and to floss between each tooth to remove any remaining debris. Flossing also helps stimulate the gums and remove bacteria.

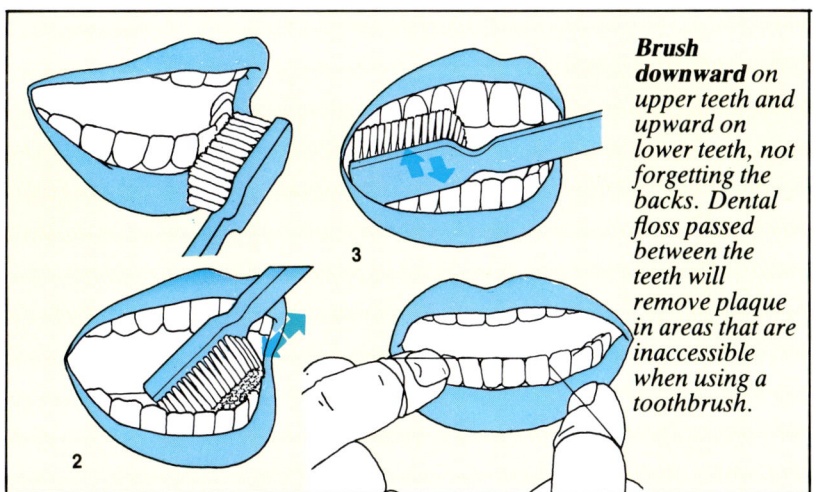

Brush downward on upper teeth and upward on lower teeth, not forgetting the backs. Dental floss passed between the teeth will remove plaque in areas that are inaccessible when using a toothbrush.

▶ *THE NOSE*

The nose is both an airway for breathing and the organ of smell. It moistens and warms the air that we breathe. The hairs and the mucous lining of the nose prevent dust and other irritants from entering the throat. The nose is made of bone and cartilage, and contains two cavities separated by a thin cartilage partition — the septum.

Fractures of the nose are a common nose injury. Since bleeding doesn't always accompany a fracture, a physician should be consulted if there is any question, especially if the swelling doesn't go down overnight. A fractured nose should be set within two weeks or it may not heal properly, giving the nose odd bumps and lumps and possibly difficulty in breathing. Although a fractured nose usually takes about six weeks to heal, the swelling may persist for six months to a year.

When the septum is crooked for some reason, it is called deviated. A deviated septum often has little to no effect on the body, but it may give the appearance of a crooked nose and sometimes creates difficulty breathing through the nose because one passageway is smaller than usual. It can be corrected with a fairly simple surgical procedure in which the deformed sections of bone and cartilage are cut away.

Rhinoplasty is another word for plastic surgery on the nose. While we all know beauty comes from within, that's sometimes hard to remember if you are dissatisfied with your appearance. The nose is one of the few parts of the body that can be modified safely and with relative ease. It may take up to a year for a restructured nose to "settle in" to its new shape.

SINUSITIS

The sinuses are air spaces lined with mucous membranes, located within the bones of the face and skull. They are connected to the nasal cavity through small openings. Their function is thought to be to lighten the weight of the skull.

Sinusitis, an inflammation of the mucous membranes that line the sinuses, is a very common condition. It can be acute (sudden, short, sharp attacks), or chronic (constant irritation). Normally, tiny hairs in the sinuses clear out mucus. When the membranes become inflamed, the hairs don't work properly and the mucus collects in the sinus cavity. Acute sinusitis tends to clear up fairly quickly. In chronic sinusitis, the lining of the sinus becomes permanently sticky and thick, blocking proper drainage.

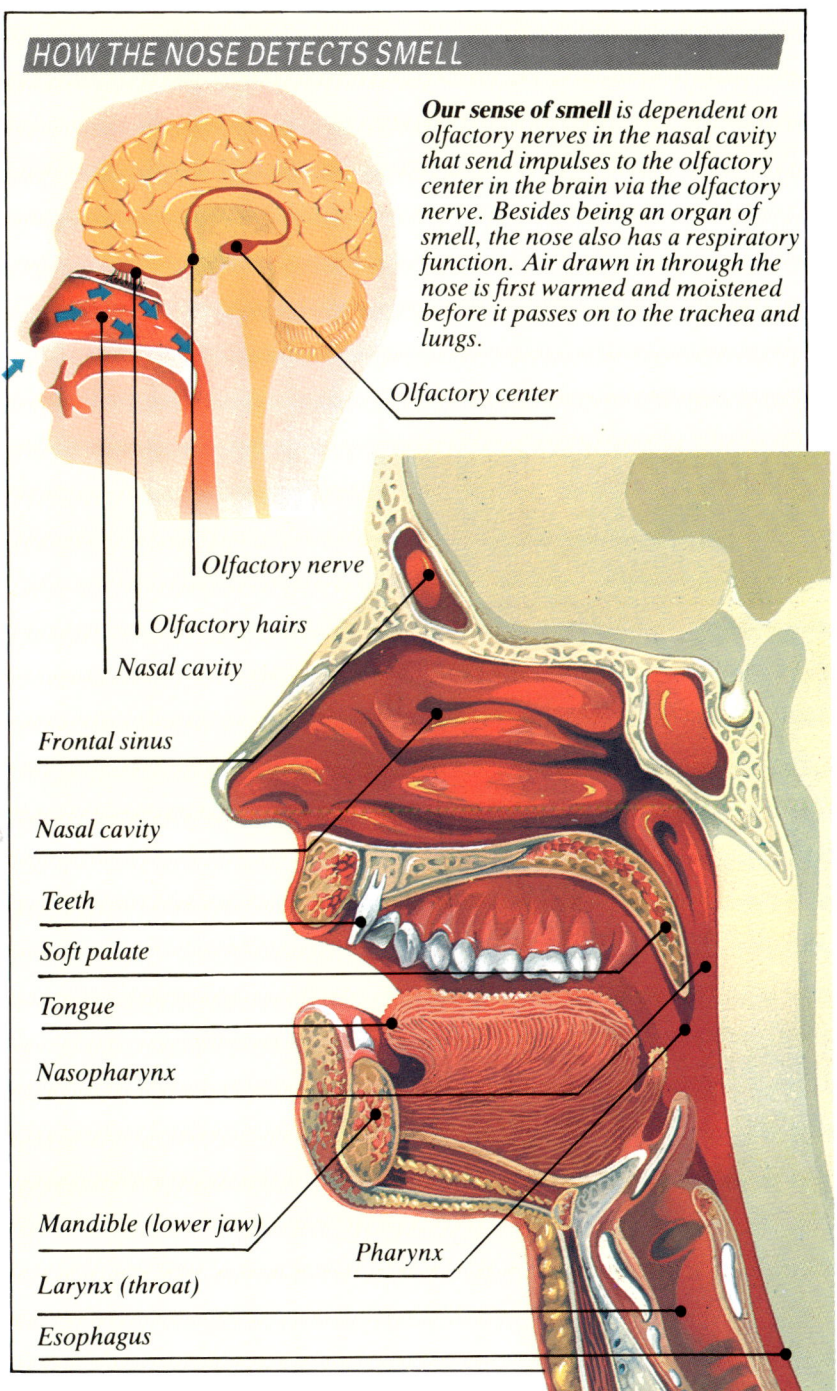

HOW THE NOSE DETECTS SMELL

Our sense of smell is dependent on olfactory nerves in the nasal cavity that send impulses to the olfactory center in the brain via the olfactory nerve. Besides being an organ of smell, the nose also has a respiratory function. Air drawn in through the nose is first warmed and moistened before it passes on to the trachea and lungs.

Olfactory center

Olfactory nerve

Olfactory hairs

Nasal cavity

Frontal sinus

Nasal cavity

Teeth

Soft palate

Tongue

Nasopharynx

Mandible (lower jaw)

Pharynx

Larynx (throat)

Esophagus

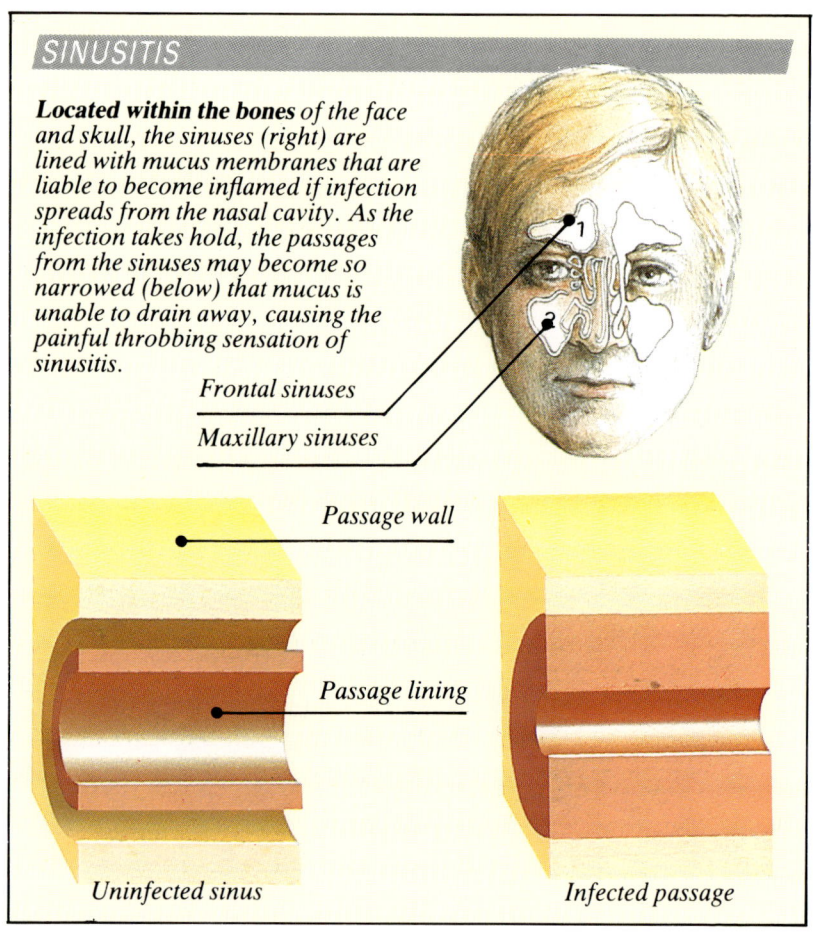

SINUSITIS

Located within the bones of the face and skull, the sinuses (right) are lined with mucus membranes that are liable to become inflamed if infection spreads from the nasal cavity. As the infection takes hold, the passages from the sinuses may become so narrowed (below) that mucus is unable to drain away, causing the painful throbbing sensation of sinusitis.

Frontal sinuses

Maxillary sinuses

Passage wall

Passage lining

Uninfected sinus

Infected passage

The symptoms of acute sinusitis may include a heavy, dull, or painful throbbing sensation around the nose and eyes, headache, and a stuffy and runny nose. The bones around the sinus may become tender to the touch. Chronic sinusitis is something many people live with without being aware of it. It can include a nose that is always blocked and stuffy, and a dull, heavy feeling in the face. People who have chronic sinusitis tend to get colds and other upper respiratory tract illnesses more easily, and they may last longer.

Acute sinusitis is thought to be caused by blowing the nose hard during a cold or flu and forcing germs into the sinuses. It can also be related to an infection of the tooth or upper jaw, or an injury or fracture of a tooth in the upper jaw or a bone surrounding the sinuses. Chronic sinusitis is thought to be caused by long-term conditions where the drainage holes into the nose are blocked, perhaps as a result of hay fever or the like. Sinusitis may be aggravated by very damp or very dry weather, very hot or very cold temperatures, and air pollution.

Treatment may include rest, use of steam and nasal sprays that shrink the mucous membranes. Sometimes aspirin will help relieve the symptoms. Nasal sprays should not be used regularly over long periods of time. In the case of an infection, antibiotics may be needed. Surgical correction is sometimes indicated in chronic problematic cases not responding to normal treatment.

NOSEBLEEDS

Nosebleeds may be caused by a variety of factors, including an injury to the nose or the base of the skull, a foreign body in the nose, operations, violent coughing, sneezing or nose blowing, nose picking, benign or malignant tumors, and weak veins in the mucous membranes of the nose. Other factors contributing to a nosebleed may be high blood presure, atmospheric changes, and excessive dry heat.

If bleeding is occurring from only one nostril, it's more likely to be from a local cause rather than from an injury. The simplest way to control a nosebleed is by applying firm, direct pressure on the side of the nose that the bleeding is coming from. Sit with the head tilted forward to keep the blood from trickling down the back of the throat, and stay sitting up to keep the head higher than the heart. Cold packs can also help stop a nosebleed. If the bleeding is coming from both nostrils or the back of the nose, emergency medical treatment may be necessary. A physician should be consulted about frequent nosebleeds.

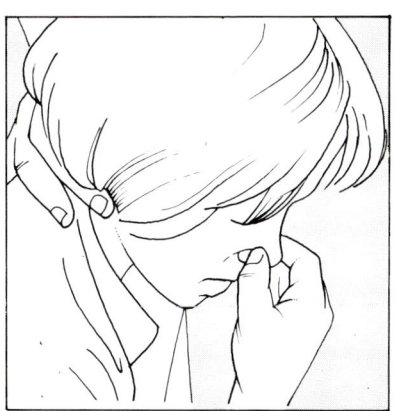

Treat a nosebleed *by pinching the nostrils closed and tilting the head forward to prevent blood trickling down the back of the throat. If the bleeding does not stop after about 10 minutes, an ice pack or cold compress applied to the nose may help. A physician should be consulted if these measures are ineffective, if bleeding is from both nostrils or if it originates from the back of the nose.*

▶ *ALLERGIES*

An allergy is an abnormal sensitivity to one or more substances. What one person is allergic to may not bother another at all. Hay fever is an allergy to plant pollens. There are also allergies to food, skin allergies, and drug allergies. Almost any substance that we inhale, swallow or touch can potentially cause an allergy. A substance that causes an allergy is called an allergen.

Sometimes a person can be exposed to a substance for months or years before an allergy to it develops. Fatigue, emotional stress, and infections can bring on an allergy. Lifestyle changes, such as moving, can bring on allergies, as can physical changes such as puberty, menopause, and pregnancy. Although allergies have a very real physical cause, they are often brought on by strong emotions such as fear, anger, and excitement.

Some of the most common allergens include the pollen of grass, trees, weeds and flowers, mold, dust, animal hair, specific foods, cosmetics, chemical dyes, and drugs. Some of the most common allergic illnesses are hay fever, asthma, hives, eczema, contact dermatitis from substances such as poison ivy, migraine headaches, and allergic rhinitis (stuffy sinuses).

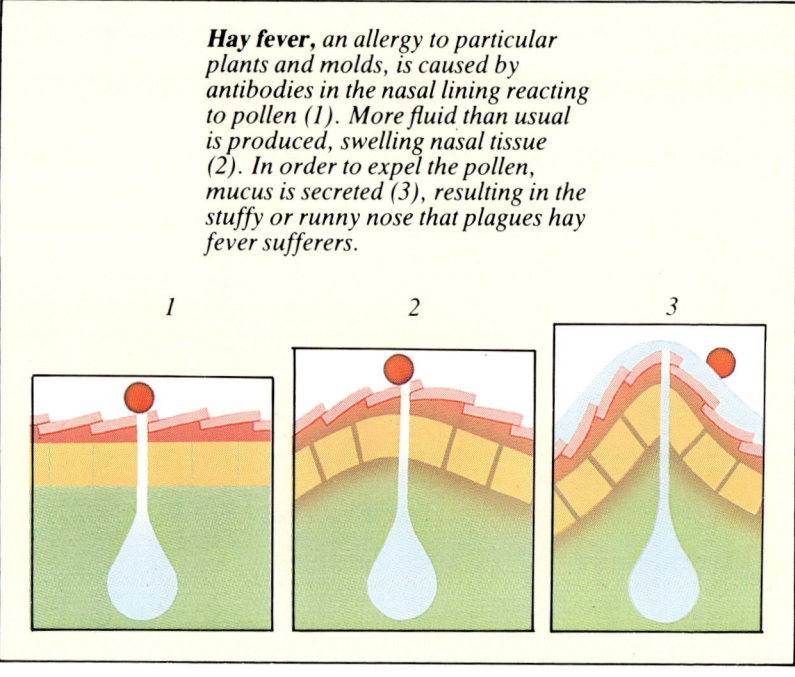

Hay fever, *an allergy to particular plants and molds, is caused by antibodies in the nasal lining reacting to pollen (1). More fluid than usual is produced, swelling nasal tissue (2). In order to expel the pollen, mucus is secreted (3), resulting in the stuffy or runny nose that plagues hay fever sufferers.*

1   *2*   *3*

The tendency to develop allergies is believed to be inherited. This means that a child whose parents have allergies is more likely to have them than one whose parents do not have allergies. If both parents are allergic, there's a fifty–fifty chance the child will be allergic. If only one parent is allergic, the chances are one in four that the child will be allergic.

Allergies rarely go away by themselves. They sometimes return after they have been treated, but more often a new sensitivity develops.

The most common symptoms of an allergic reaction are sneezing, shortness of breath, wheezing, a stuffy and runny nose, itching skin, hives, and swellings. Less common symptoms include headaches, severe rashes, diarrhea, vomiting, and muscle cramps. Allergies can become serious when they create other illnesses. For example, hay fever can become sinusitis or asthma. Allergies are rarely fatal, though an extreme reaction, usually to a drug, can be fatal. Though it is very rare, deaths have been caused by the stings of wasps, bees, and yellow jackets.

Plant allergies are among the most common, and are usually seasonal. Hay fever is a specific respiratory allergy caused by plants and molds. People allergic to tree pollens suffer most in the spring when the trees are in blossom. Molds tend to appear in the summer during hot, humid weather, and grasses pollinate in late spring and early summer. Most people who have hay fever get it in late summer and early fall when weeds such as ragweeds are pollinating. Most pollen is released between 6 A.M. and 1 P.M., so hay fever sufferers can find some relief by staying inside during those hours.

The simplest cure for an allergy is to remove the cause. This may mean an animal, and for some people it actually means moving to a different environment. A series of injections over a period of months to desensitize the person can also be a permanent cure for a specific allergy.

Finding out specifically what is causing an allergy can be a real challenge to a physician, and yet it is the key step to treating it. The diagnosis is made through a careful study of the patient's lifestyle and habits, and from there picking specific substances to be tested out of an almost infinite number. The tests are made by injecting extracts of the substance under the skin, which will show evidence of sensitivity with a red welt or swelling. Blood tests can also reveal specific allergens.

FOOD ALLERGIES

With each passing year, scientists and researchers isolate more and more foods that may be responsible for allergies ranging from mild

HAY FEVER

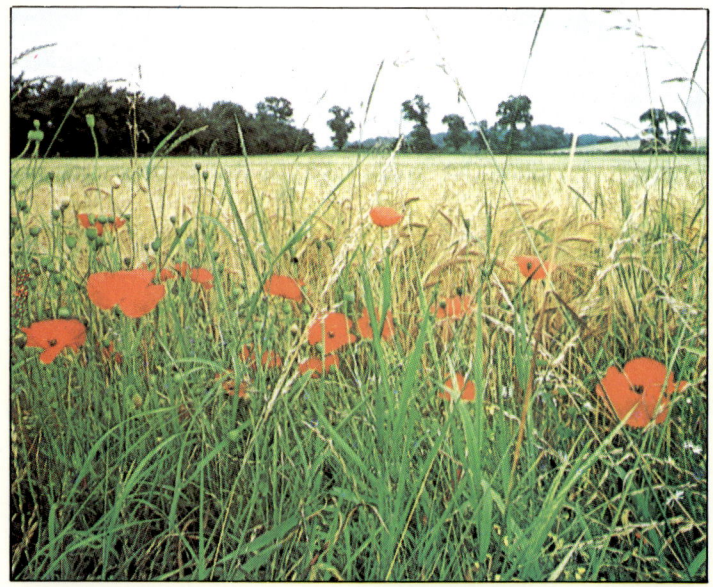

Seed plants (top) produce the pollens to which sufferers of hay fever are allergic. Symptoms include repeated sneezing, a congested or runny nose, itchy skin and streaming eyes.

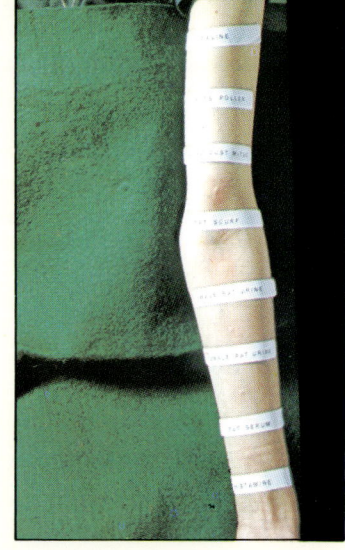

Tests (above) can determine allergen sensitivity.

to severe. It is also increasingly accepted in the medical community that some foods may create low-profile allergies that cause generalized illnesses such as arthritis, sinusitis, headaches, fatigue, and muscle weakness. More obvious signs of a food allergy may include belching, nausea, vomiting, constipation, diarrhea, stomach cramps, and canker sores in the mouth.

Allergies to food are identified by putting the patient on a very restricted diet for a few days. Then, a few at a time, "suspect" foods are added to the diet, and the patient is observed closely for a reaction. The allergic reaction can take place right away, or may be delayed for a day or so. Oddly enough, the foods that are most suspect as allergens are the ones eaten habitually — every day without fail. A simple test can be done at home simply by eliminating those foods for a day, reintroducing them one at a time, and observing how the body reacts. The most common reactions to mild food allergies may include increased pulse rate and nausea.

Some of the most common food allergens include sugar, chocolate, milk and other dairy products, wheat, corn, red meat, citrus fruits, melons, and the nightshade family of plants, which includes tomatoes, potatoes, peppers and eggplants. Shellfish and strawberries have been known to cause sudden and acute allergic reactions.

Food allergies are treated by simply eliminating the offending food from the diet. Often a food allergen can be gradually reintroduced into the diet after a period of time. An acute food allergy can be treated with antihistamines.

SKIN ALLERGIES

Children tend to have skin allergies more than adults. The most common skin allergy is known as contact dermatitis, which simply means a skin reaction that might include a rash, swelling, or bumps. The rashes caused by poison ivy, poison oak, and poison sumac are a form of contact dermatitis. Other skin allergies include eczema and hives.

The symptoms of contact dermatitis are itching and redness of the skin, swelling, blisters, crusting, scaling, and oozing. It can occur in one spot or cover the entire body. Contact dermatitis is most often caused by medicines, clothing, chemicals, cosmetics, deodorants, plant oils, plastics, dyes, and foods. It can be treated with antihistamine drugs and skin ointments to relieve the symptoms, but removing the cause is the best medicine.

Eczema is a specific type of dermatitis. Its symptoms include scaling, flaking, and blistering. It is almost always caused by a food allergen.

Hives are usually caused by foods or drugs. They are identified by large, red, and frequently intensely itchy patches of skin. Hives usually occur around the face or the back but can appear on any part of the body. Shellfish, strawberries, highly seasoned foods, and aspirin are the most frequent causes of hives.

DRUG ALLERGIES

Drug allergies are often severe and sometimes fatal. The symptoms can range from a runny and stuffy nose or skin rash, to asthma attacks or seizures. The long-term treatment for a drug allergy is to not take it again. In severe reactions antihistamines or steroid drugs may help. It's always important to inform medical personnel of any drug allergies you may have. If you have a severe, potentially life-threatening drug allergy, it's wise to wear a "medic alert" bracelet that details the problem.

INSECT ALLERGIES

Many people are allergic to the stings of wasps, hornets, bees, and yellow jackets. Some develop a sensitivity that increases each time they are stung, until the allergy becomes life-threatening. Common sense is the best way to avoid insect stings. Many people who are extremely sensitive to insect stings carry a kit with them when they are outdoors that includes drugs to immediately counteract the allergic reaction.

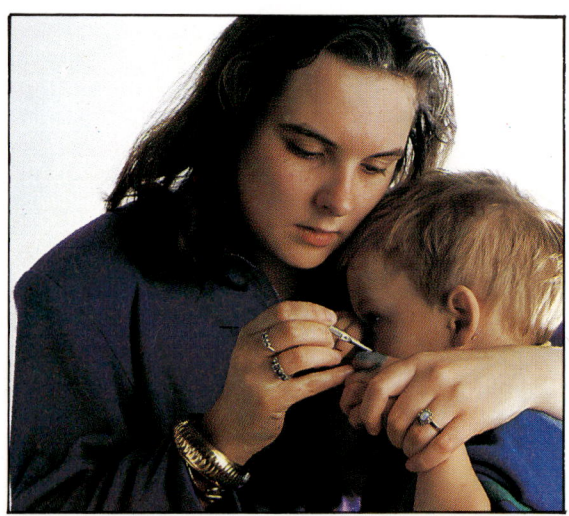

Locate the *insect sting if it is present and mark its position with a colored food dye as accurately as possible. Remove the sting with a pair of tweezers that have been sterilized. Then apply an antihistimine cream or calamine lotion.*

▶ THE EARS

The ears are the sensory organs that allow us to hear sounds. Sound waves enter through the external ear canal and strike the eardrum, causing it to vibrate. The vibrations of the eardrum are transmitted to three tiny bones (the ossicles) which are found on the inner part of the drum. The ossicles vibrate and transmit impulses to the inner ear. The inner ear is filled with fluid and surrounded by a membrane. The vibrations of the ossicles are transmitted through the membrane and fluid of the inner ear to special nerve endings. These nerve endings are in turn connected to a special auditory nerve; this transmits the sound impulses to the brain, where we interpret them as sound, or hearing.

The middle ear, which is located behind the eardrum and houses the ossicles, is connected to the throat by the Eustachian tubes, which equalize air pressure in the ear. When you feel your ears pop in an elevator or in an airplane, that is the middle ear at work. The popping can also be created when mucus blocks the Eustachian tubes. Yawning or chewing gum often helps the middle ear equalize air pressure.

The inner ear provides us with our sense of balance and our sense of gravity — our perception of "which way is up."

How accurately we hear depends on many factors and can vary tremendously from person to person. Hearing can be painlessly tested by an audiologist with a device called an audiometer, which can accurately show the range of hearing in each ear. Someone with a hearing loss may be fitted with a hearing aid. These can be extremely effective in restoring much lost hearing, particularly in the case of the nerve deafness that is almost inevitable as we grow older. The technology of hearing aids is improving constantly, and most are quite comfortable and inconspicuous.

COMMON EAR PROBLEMS

Ear wax is an important part of normal ear functioning, as it lubricates and protects the eardrum and the skin in the ear passage. Excess wax in the ear is a common problem. For reasons that are not known, the wax glands in the ear sometimes secrete too much wax, and this creates a blockage of the ear canal, which can result in loss of hearing. Sometimes the wax lodges up against the eardrum, which creates a more profound loss of hearing.

Sometimes the water of a shower or swim softens wax in the ear canal; as it dries and hardens, it obstructs the canal. The symptoms

THE STRUCTURE OF THE EAR

Eardrum

Semicircular canals

Ossicles

Eustachian tube

Cochlea

External auditory canal (conveys vibrations of sound to eardrum)

Auricle (collects sound waves)

Auditory nerve

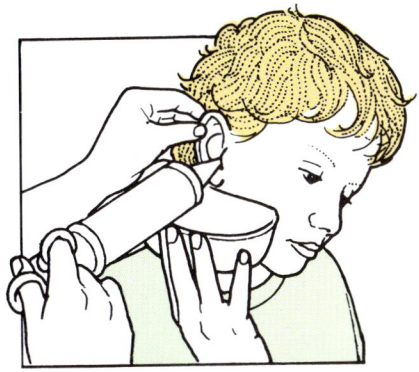

Although it seems unlikely, *wax is in fact secreted by the ear to cleanse it. Occasionally, the wax may harden and accumulate, blocking the ear canal. A ringing in the ears, earache and partial deafness may all indicate that this is the case and that the affected ear needs syringing (left).*

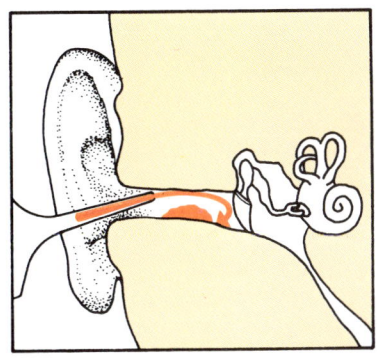

When a physician syringes *an ear that has become blocked by wax, he or she points the syringe (filled with warm water) at the top of the ear canal, rather than directly into it, to flush out the blockage (left). Because the ear canal is easily damaged, you should never try self-treatment by inserting anything into the ear yourself, but always seek medical advice.*

of excess ear wax are loss of hearing, irritation in the ear, and sometimes a discharge of pus if infection is present.

Wax that is lodged inside the ear can sometimes be removed with ear drops. If that doesn't work within a few days, a physician should remove the wax, usually with a warm-water syringe or a vacuum suction device. The old saying still applies: Do not put anything smaller than your elbow in your ear!

Perforation or puncturing of the eardrum is one of the most common ear ailments. This is a break in the eardrum caused by infection or injury — usually by sticking something you shouldn't in your ear. The symptoms of a perforated eardrum can include pain, loss of or altered hearing, dizziness, nausea, and blood in the ear canal. If there is an infection, the symptoms can be a sharp, stabbing pain, a sensation of fullness in the ear, ringing in the ear and a fever.

A small perforation in the eardrum usually heals itself with time. Antibiotics may be prescribed by a doctor if infection is present. A major perforation of the ear can require extremely delicate reconstructive surgery.

Otitis media is a middle ear infection, usually caused by the spread of infection up through the Eustachian tubes during a cold, flu or throat infection. (The Eustachian tubes connect the middle ear with the back of the throat.) Symptoms may include pain in the ear, hearing loss, fever and a red, swollen eardrum. If the eardrum has been ruptured, there may be a discharge of pus into the external ear canal. Though a middle ear infection can be treated with antibiotics, the best treatment is prevention. This means taking care of colds, flu, sinus infections, sore throats, and swollen adenoids or tonsils. It also helps to blow the nose gently so that the mucus is not forced from the sinuses back into the Eustachian tubes. Avoid sniffing mucus back into the sinuses if possible, as this too can force it into the Eustachian tubes.

Ménière's disease is a disorder of the inner ear that tends to come and go suddenly. The symptoms may include sudden vertigo or loss of balance, buzzing and ringing in the ears, headache and vomiting, vision disturbance, and impairment of hearing. Its cause is not

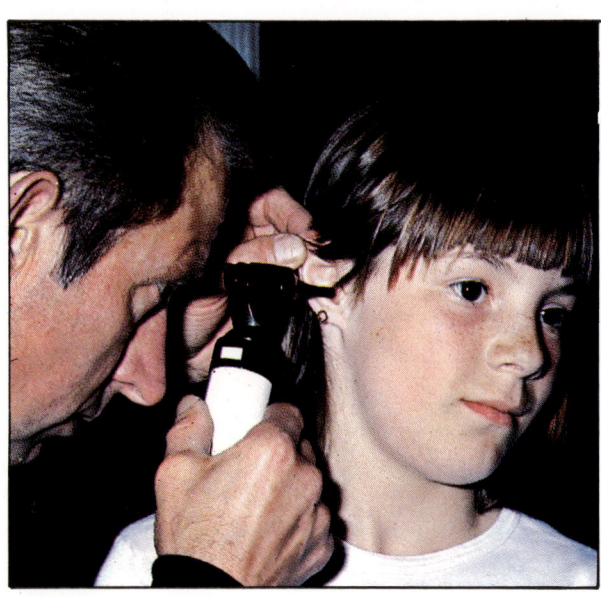

If an ear infection or disorder seems to be indicated by the patient's symptoms, a physician will confirm his diagnosis by using an otoscope (which projects light) to examine the inner structures of the ear. The diagram shows how the eardrum appears through an otoscope — a perforation is revealed clearly as a nonreflective hole.

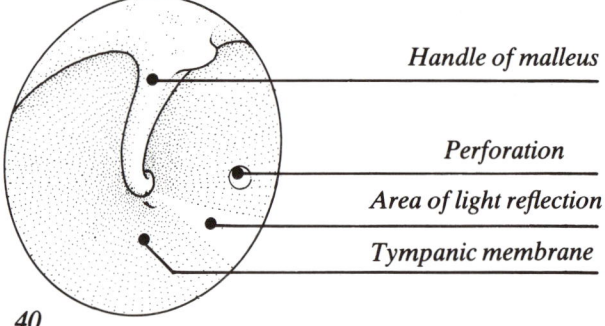

Handle of malleus

Perforation

Area of light reflection

Tympanic membrane

known and treatment is uncertain. A low-sodium diet and a vitamin supplement of nicotinic acid is often recommended. In severe cases surgery may be needed to reduce the pressure in the inner ear.

Tinnitus, or ringing in the ears, can be caused by high blood pressure and overdoses of antibiotics or aspirin. It can also be associated with diseases of the ear.

Deafness can be caused by any interference with the normal functioning of the ear assembly, from the external ear canal to the auditory nerve leading to the brain. Deafness is often caused by a failure of some part of the ear to develop properly before birth, and can also be related to a dysfunction of the central nervous system. Deafness may be caused temporarily or permanently by disease, drugs, occupational hazards such as overexposure to loud noise, tumors, and foreign bodies in the ears. Deafness can often be treated by hearing aids, medication, and in some cases, surgery.

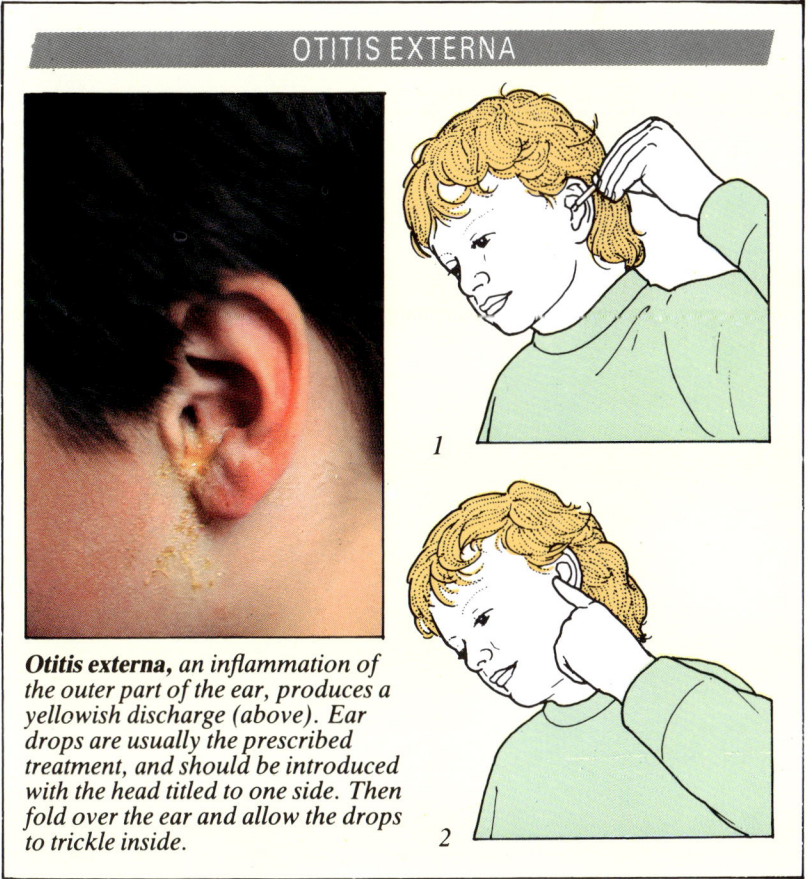

OTITIS EXTERNA

Otitis externa, an inflammation of the outer part of the ear, produces a yellowish discharge (above). Ear drops are usually the prescribed treatment, and should be introduced with the head titled to one side. Then fold over the ear and allow the drops to trickle inside.

1

2

▶ THE EYES

The eyes are the sensory organ that allow us to see the world around us. Your eyes work much the same way a camera does. The lens is located toward the front of the eye; it is held in place by the ciliary muscle and protected by the cornea. Light enters the eye through the cornea or outer covering of the eye, and goes through the iris, which is the colored part of the eye, and the pupil, which is the round black spot in the middle of the eye.

Tiny muscles in the eye contract or expand to change the size of the pupil, and thus the amount of light that passes through. As the light passes through the cornea and lens it bends and strikes the retina at the back of the eye. The retina, made up of light-sensitive "rods" and "cones," receives the light and transforms it into encoded impulses which are passed, via nerve fibers, to the optic nerve and the brain. The rods in the retina are sensitive to gray and white light, while the cones pick up reds, blues, and greens. Two sources of nourishment and protection for the eye are the aqueous humor, a layer of watery fluid between the cornea and the lens, and the vitreous humor, which is a transparent, jellylike substance that makes up most of the eyeball.

NEARSIGHTEDNESS

Nearsightedness, or myopia, means that the vision is better for near objects than objects that are far away. It is caused when the eyeball is slightly longer than normal, causing the lens of the eye to focus in front of the retina, blurring everything but near-distance objects. About one-third of all the people who wear glasses are nearsighted. The condition can be corrected with a concave lens in the glasses. Nearsightedness is generally inherited. It sometimes gets worse with age because the eyeball tends to get larger while the rest of the optical system remains the same.

A new surgical procedure called radial keratotomy changes the curvature of the cornea by making tiny incisions around the eyeball. The procedure is new and somewhat controversial, and is not generally recommended except for some cases of extreme nearsightedness.

Of all the body's organs, the eye's intricate structure (right) makes it the most complex and also the most prone to disorder.

STRUCTURE OF THE EYE

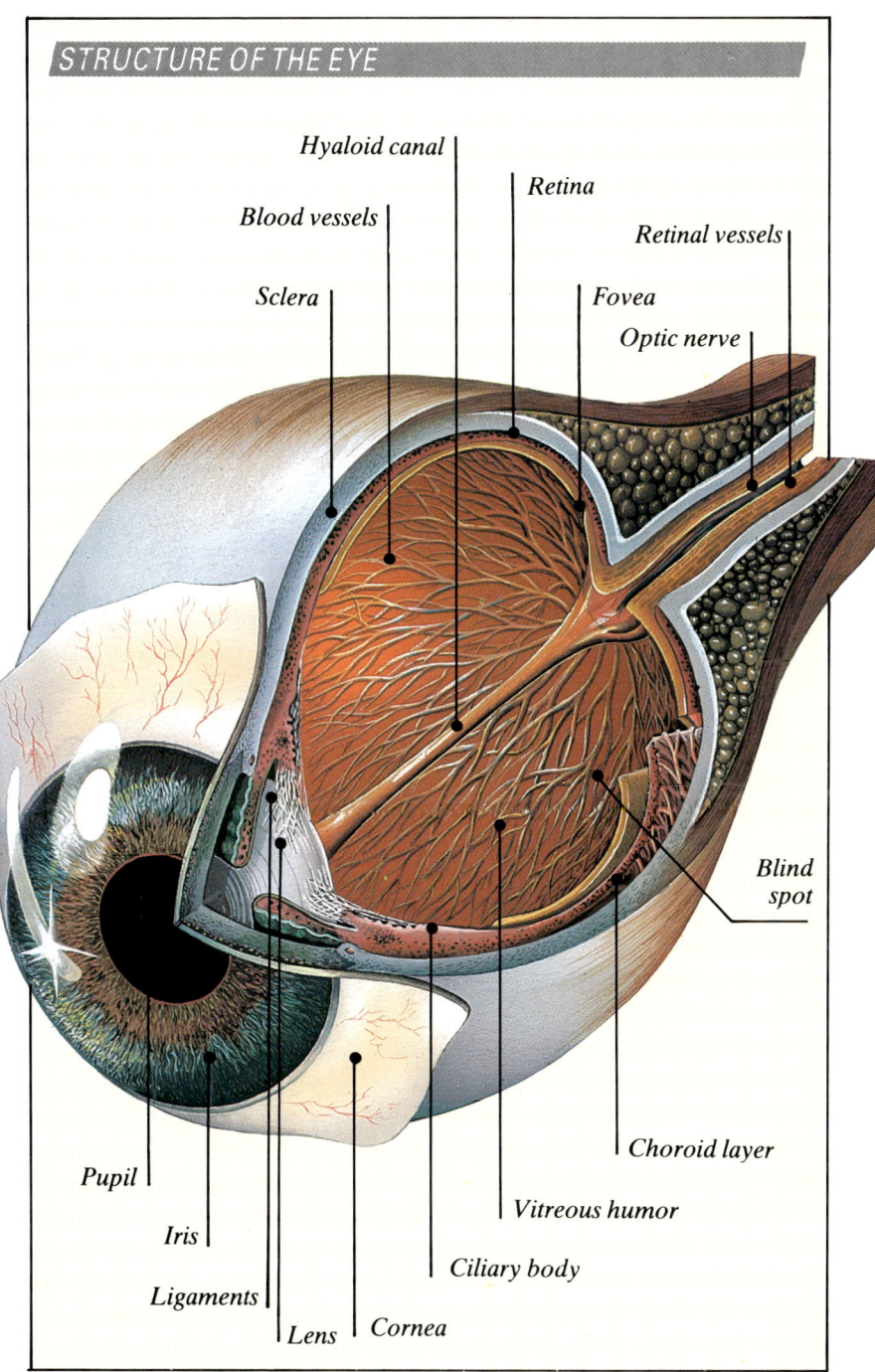

Hyaloid canal

Blood vessels

Retina

Sclera

Retinal vessels

Fovea

Optic nerve

Blind spot

Choroid layer

Vitreous humor

Pupil

Iris

Ciliary body

Ligaments

Lens

Cornea

Nearsightedness, or *myopia, occurs when the eyeball is slightly longer than normal, with the result that the lens of the eye focuses in front of the retina and only near objects can be seen clearly.*

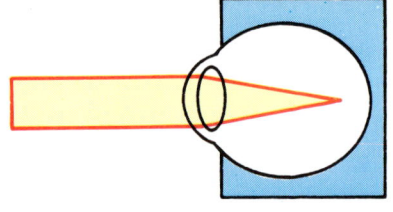

Glasses fitted with concave lenses correct the condition to give a normal range of vision.

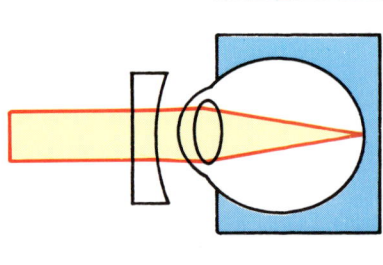

In farsightedness, or *hypermetropia, the lens of the eye focuses behind the retina, blurring everything but distant objects. It is caused by the eyeball being shorter than normal.*

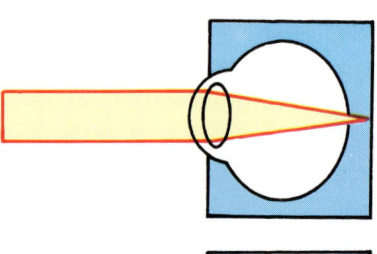

Glasses fitted with convex lenses correct the defect and restore the full range of vision.

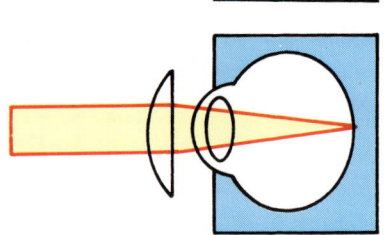

FARSIGHTEDNESS

Farsightedness, or hypermetropia, means that vision is better for far objects than for objects that are near. In this case the eyeball is slightly shorter than normal and the lens of the eye focuses images "behind" the retina. About one-third of all those who wear glasses are farsighted. The condition can be corrected with a convex lens. Farsightedness can also get worse with age, as the lens of the eye becomes more rigid and the eye muscles don't compensate as well.

ASTIGMATISM

Astigmatism is a defect in the curvature of the cornea and/or lens of the eye. This creates an imbalance that prevents light rays from hitting the retina at a point of common focus. The symptoms of astigmatism can be constant eyestrain and blurred vision. The condition can be easily helped with a corrective lens.

CONJUNCTIVITIS

Conjunctivitis is an inflammation of the conjunctiva, which is the membrane covering the eyeball and the inside of the eyelids. It rarely causes permanent damage to the eye. The symptoms are redness, itching, burning, tearing, swelling of the eyelid, and a gritty feeling underneath the eyelids. If there is infection present there may be a discharge of pus. Conjunctivitis may be caused by injury, infection, allergy, or excessive exposure to sun, wind, dust, and air pollution. The common bacteria streptococcus can cause

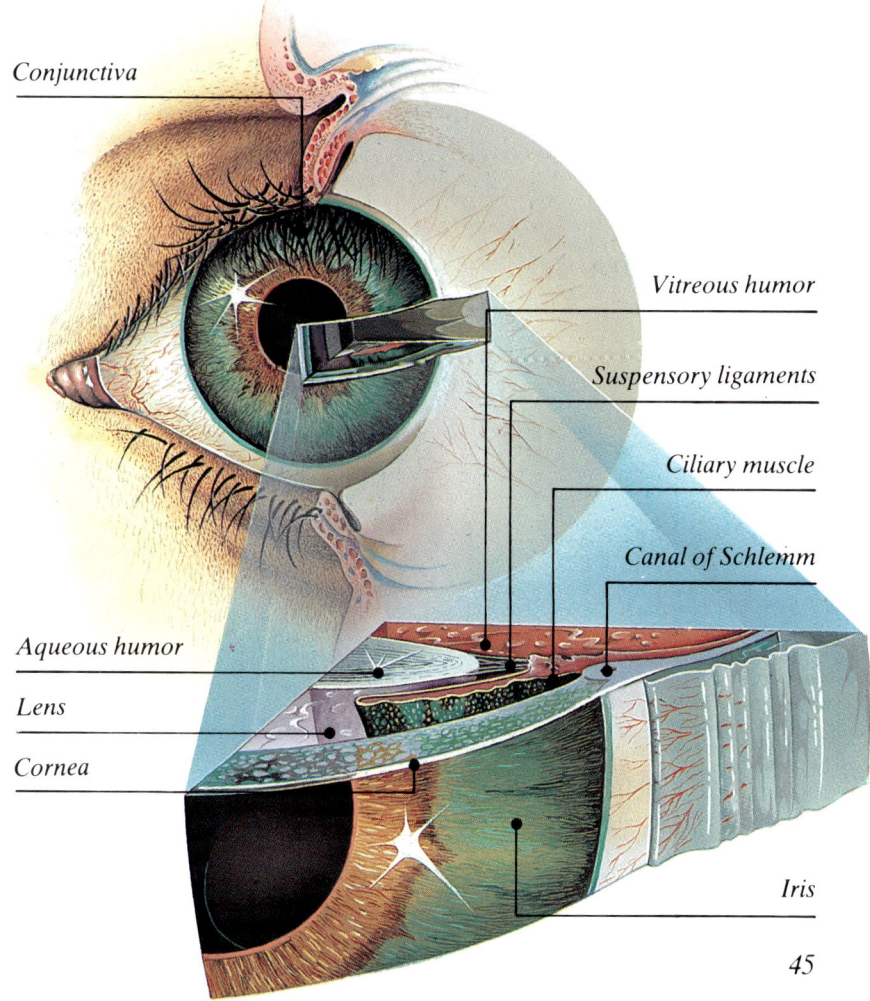

Conjunctiva

Vitreous humor

Suspensory ligaments

Ciliary muscle

Canal of Schlemm

Aqueous humor

Lens

Cornea

Iris

conjunctivitis through infection. Eye make-up can become contaminated by bacteria that can cause an eye infection.

For conjunctivitis caused by injury or exposure, treatment may include mildly astringent eyedrops, frequent eye baths, cold compresses, and dark glasses if there is a sensitivity to the light. It's very important to keep the eye area clean. Eye make-up should be avoided until the condition has cleared up.

The infectious type of conjunctivitis can be treated with antibiotic drops. Allergic conjunctivitis may be treated with antihistamine drops. Infectious types of conjunctivitis can be contagious, so it's important not to share towels, soap, pillowcases, or anything else that comes into contact with the eyes. "Pinkeye" is a contagious type of infectious conjunctivitis.

GLAUCOMA

Glaucoma is a condition of the eye in which fluid builds in the eyeball and creates pressure. If not treated, the pressure can damage the retina and the optic nerve, causing full or partial blindness. Glaucoma usually occurs after the age of 40, and can be inherited. The presence of glaucoma may not be noticed until the vision in both eyes is impaired. Symptoms leading up to glaucoma can include headaches, misty vision, loss of peripheral vision, and rainbow borders around lights. When glaucoma is acute the symptoms may include severe pain, extreme sensitivity to light, redness, blurring of the vision, and nausea. The test for glaucoma is very simple and should be performed at the time of an eye check-up or exam. Glaucoma is usually treated with medication.

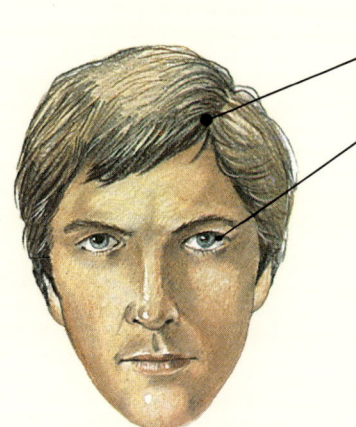

Headaches

Eyesight impairment, pain and misty vision

Pressure in the eyeball *through the build-up of fluid is the cause of glaucoma, a condition which may lead to blindness if it is left untreated and continued pressure damages the retina or optic nerve. Any unusual headaches or impairment of vision should therefore be reported to a physician at once. If caught early enough, glaucoma is normally easily cured with drugs.*

CATARACTS

A cataract is a clouding of the lens of the eye, preventing light from entering and decreasing vision. The symptoms including blurring or dimming of the vision which can't be corrected with glasses, double vision, and a milky or whitish substance on the pupil of the eye. It's not known exactly what causes cataracts, but scientists speculate that they can be associated with diabetes, glandular disorders, infection of the eyeball, radiation, drugs, and injury to the lens of the eye. Cataracts are very common in the elderly. They are most often treated with a fairly simple and routine surgical procedure, with a good recovery rate.

EYE CARE

● An *optometrist* is trained to recognize eye diseases and prescribe glasses.
● An *ophthalmologist* is a doctor trained to diagnose and treat eye diseases and perform eye surgery.
● An *optician* makes and fits corrective lenses for eyeglasses and contact lenses.

Most people should have an eye check-up every one or two years. Those over 65 years of age should have their vision checked yearly.

Consult an eye doctor if:
● There is a change in vision, such as blurring or double vision.
● If the cornea may be cut or scratched.
● If styes or cysts appear on the eyelid.
● If the edges of the eyelids or lashes turn in or out, or cause irritation.
● If there is pain, redness, or inflammation in any part of the eye that is severe or lasts for more than a few days.

EYE PROTECTION

Wear goggles when:
● Working with chemicals or materials that may spray in the face.
● Playing sports where there's a high possibility of being hit in the face, such as racquetball, squash, or fencing.

If there is a foreign body in the eye do *not* rub the eye! Blink rapidly to increase the production of tears; gently pull the upper lid over the lower lid and hold it there for a few seconds, or bathe the eye in clean water. If chemicals get into the eyes, follow the instructions on the container or bathe the eye thoroughly in cold water. See an eye doctor immediately.

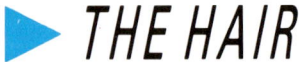

THE HAIR

Healthy, shiny, bouncy hair is, believe it or not, dead. The root of the hair is alive and grows, but the hair itself is dead, just as your fingernails are. The roots are small, buried sacs in the skin, known as hair follicles. They are nourished through the blood vessels and fat glands in the scalp. Each follicle lives for two to three years, and then the hair stops growing. When a new hair begins to grow in, the old hair is shed. Since each hair follicle grows at a different rate, only a few hairs are in the process of being shed at any given time.

DANDRUFF

Dandruff is a scalp condition in which flakes and scales of skin appear in the hair. The flaking and scaling of skin on the scalp is actually quite a normal process. When it becomes noticeable, as with dandruff, it is usually due to a much higher rate of cell turnover than usual. Dandruff can also be created by a disorder of the fat glands that nourish the hair. Dandruff is not contagious.

The best remedy for a slight dandruff problem is to purchase a dandruff shampoo containing zinc pyrithione. Those who tend to get dandruff should avoid brushing or combing the scalp too vigorously or roughly, and avoid scratching the scalp. When shampooing the hair, avoid over-massaging the scalp. Dandruff is often an indication that the scalp needs a rest.

A simple herbal treatment for dandruff is as follows: Boil four tablespoons of dried thyme leaves in two cups of water for ten minutes. It should boil down to about one cup. Strain the thyme out and let the remaining fluid cool. After shampooing the hair, pour the thyme water over the damp hair, gently comb it through, and let the hair dry. The thyme water doesn't need to be rinsed out until the next time the hair is shampooed.

Long hair (right) needs particular care because the ends tend to be brittle. Avoid using a blow dryer or hot rollers too often and allow the hair to dry naturally as frequently as you can. When brushing long hair, untangle knots at the ends first, then gradually work up to the scalp.

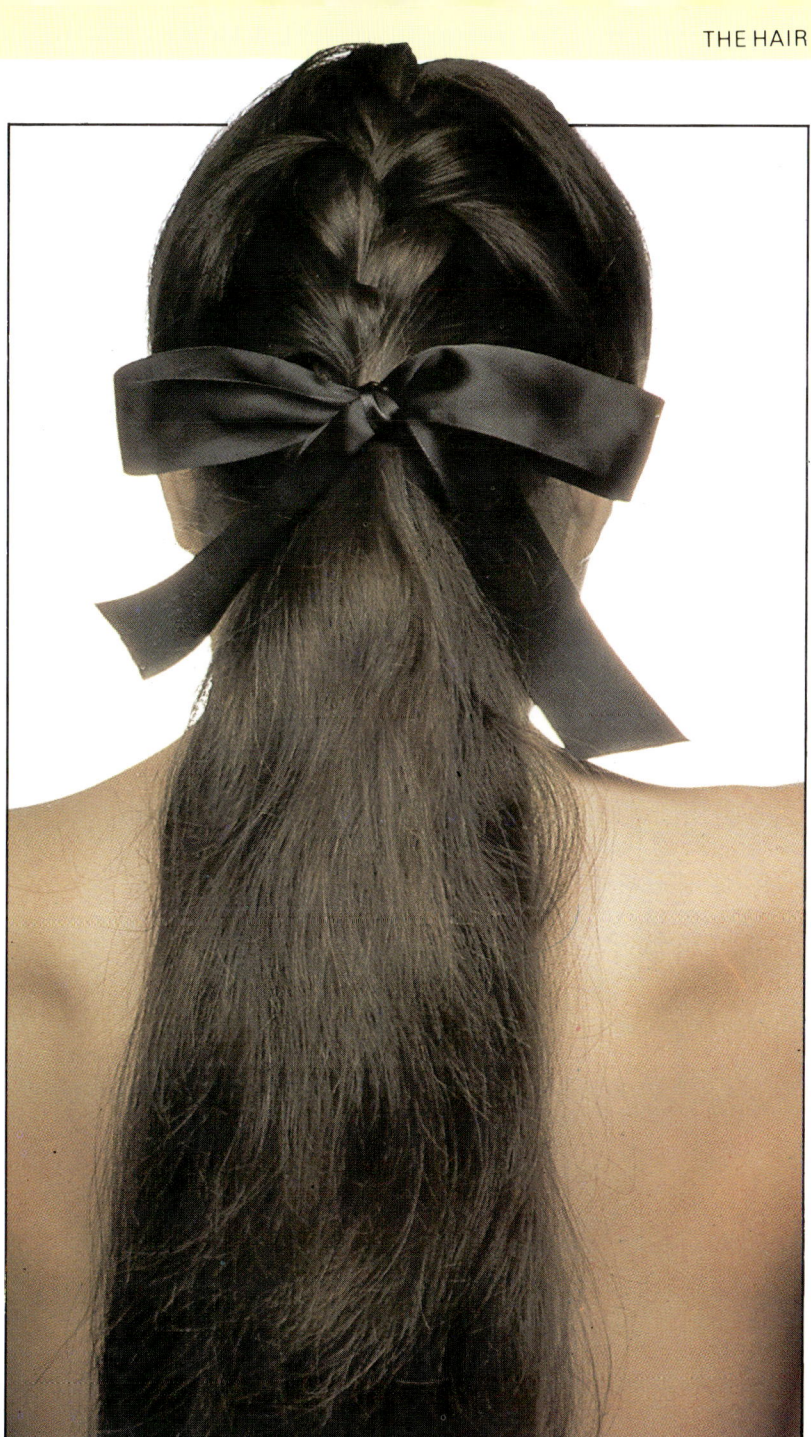

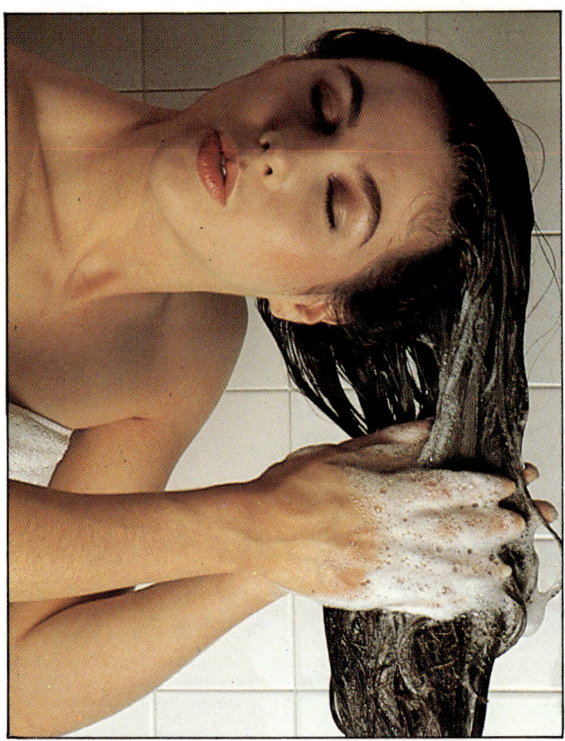

Choose a shampoo *suitable for your hair type and wash your hair as often as you think it needs it. Most hair, but especially treated hair — hair that has been colored or permed — benefits from a conditioner applied afterward.*

SHAMPOO

Hair tends to fall into three broad categories: oily, dry, and normal. Shampoo is made for all types of hair. The main ingredient in shampoo is detergent, which is designed to wash out grease and dust in the hair. How often a person shampoos his or her hair is usually determined by the environment, how oily or dry the hair is, and individual styling needs. Conditioner is especially helpful for hair that has been treated in any way, such as coloring and perming.

Frequent coloring, bleaching, and permanents can damage hair. There are shampoos and conditioners made especially for treated hair, which can be helpful.

CARING FOR THE HAIR AND SCALP

Hair looks its best when the dead, split ends are trimmed frequently. Use a wide-tooth comb or brush for untangling hair, because a fine-tooth comb tends to pull hair out. When brushing long hair, avoid tugging on it by holding it at the scalp. When possible, towel-dry the hair rather than blow-drying it. The constant use of hair dryers and hot rollers can make the hair dry and brittle.

The sun can damage treated hair, so it's best to wear a hat over hair that has been colored or permed. A gentle scalp massage can be very good for the hair because it can increase the blood circulation in the scalp.

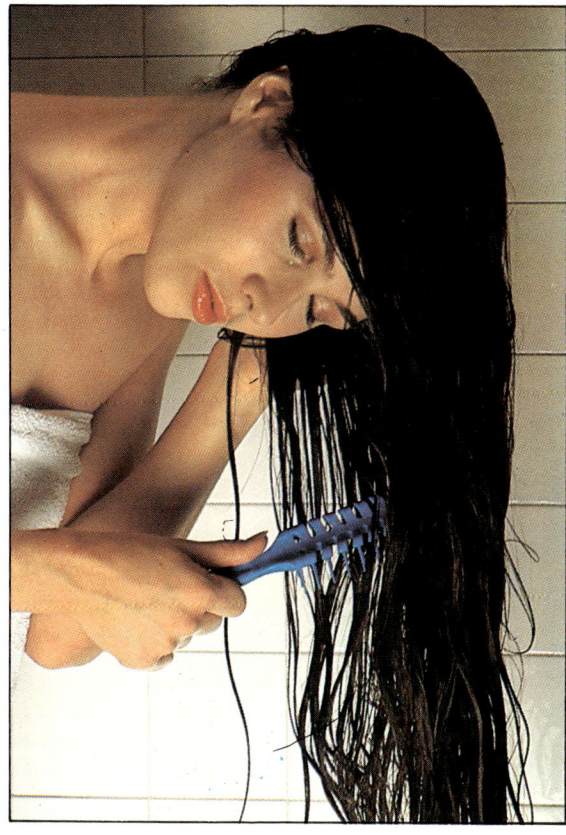

Wet hair is much more fragile than dry and brushing it can easily lead to split ends or cause ends to break. Always use a wide-tooth comb to untangle wet hair, taking a small section at a time.

ELECTROLYSIS

Electrolysis is a professional procedure used to remove unwanted hair from the body. It is most commonly used for unwanted facial hair on women. During the procedure, a tiny needle is inserted into the hair follicle, and an electric current is passed through the needle. This destroys the root of the hair, and the electrologist removes it. If done properly, electrolysis should be safe and permanent. Always have a very small patch of skin tested first to determine if the skin can tolerate the procedure.

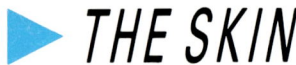 *THE SKIN*

The skin is the largest organ in the body. Most adults have about 20 square feet of skin of their body. The skin has many functions. It protects the internal organs and creates structure around the bones and muscles.

One of the most important functions of the skin is to regulate body temperature and fluids. We lose about a pint of fluid a day through perspiration alone, which underscores the importance of drinking a lot of fluids. Drinking six to eight cups of water a day can play a major role in keeping the skin healthy. Drinking water assists the body in cleansing internal tissues and removing waste materials.

Other keys to healthy-looking skin are eating a balanced and nutritious diet, getting plenty of sleep and exercise (but not too much), fresh air, and at least 30 minutes of natural daylight per day. Stress can also affect the skin. Deep-breathing exercises combined with relaxation techniques such as yoga, meditation, and creative visualization can help ease stress (these techniques are discussed later).

THE FACE NEEDS SPECIAL SKIN CARE

The skin of the face needs special care because it is especially sensitive, and tends to be exposed to the elements more than the rest of the body.

For women, it's important to remove make-up every evening with soap or a cleanser that's right for your individual skin type. In dry climates many women use a moisturizer on their skin. Prolonged exposure to the sun can cause premature aging of the skin.

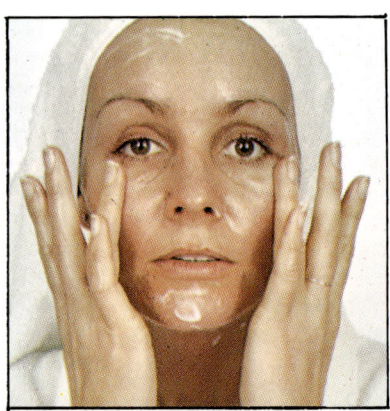

Moisturizing the face not only helps to keep skin supple, but also provides a protective barrier against the drying effects of the elements and the environment.

STRUCTURE OF THE SKIN

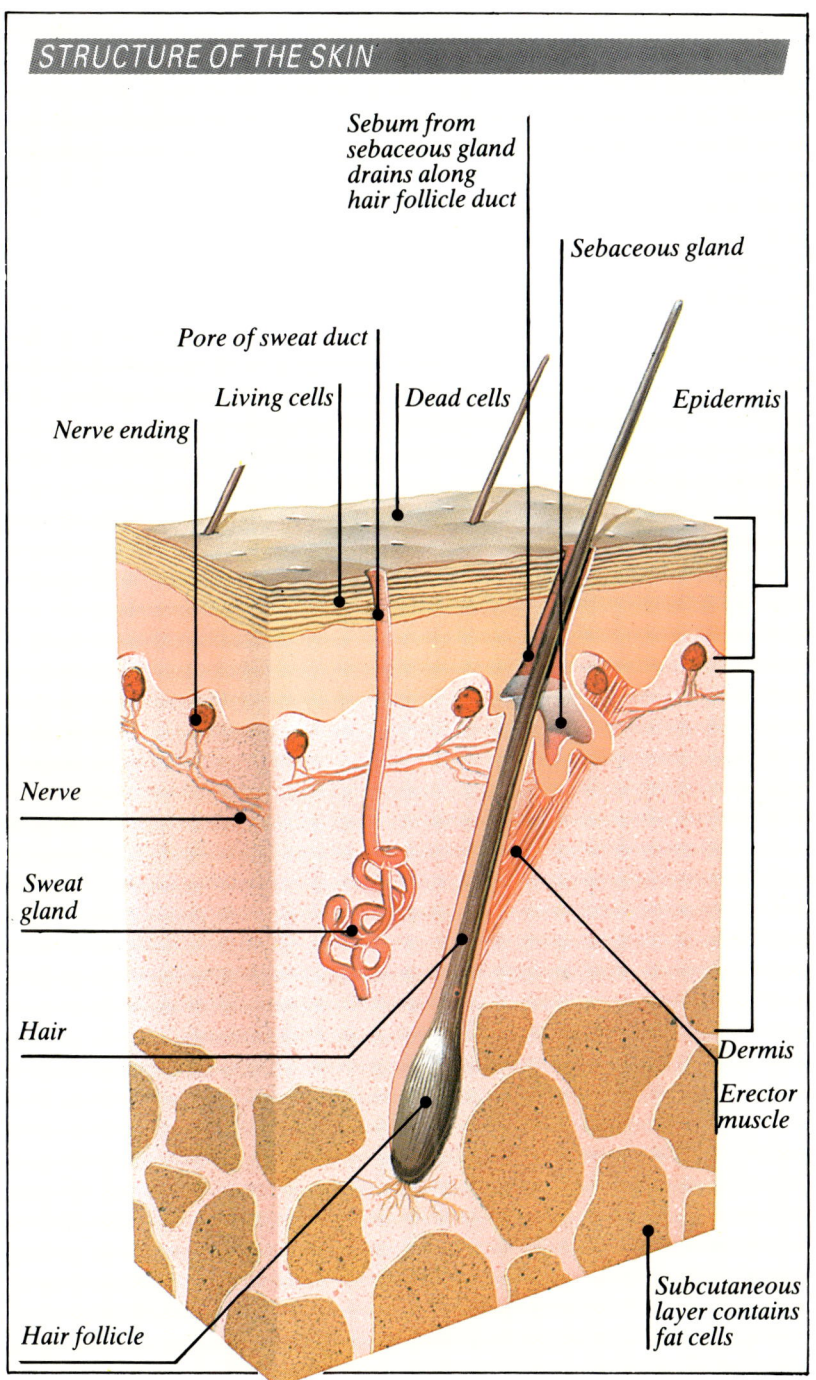

Sebum from sebaceous gland drains along hair follicle duct

Sebaceous gland

Pore of sweat duct

Living cells

Dead cells

Epidermis

Nerve ending

Nerve

Sweat gland

Hair

Dermis

Erector muscle

Hair follicle

Subcutaneous layer contains fat cells

Few adolescents *avoid the occurrence of acne after the onset of puberty. To avoid damaging the skin, and to prevent secondary infection, spots should not be squeezed, but allowed to heal naturally. Regularly washing the skin, perhaps with an acne preparation, and the avoidance of greasy foods are the best preventive measures.*

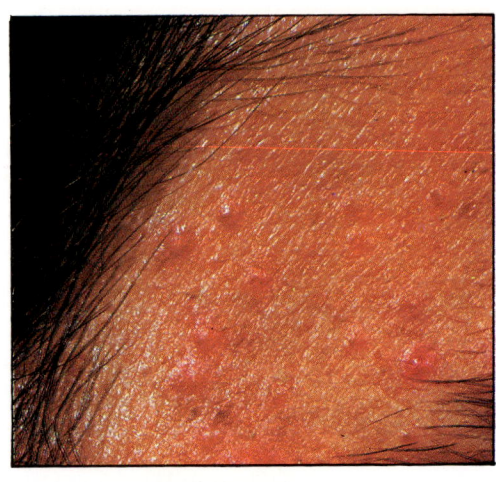

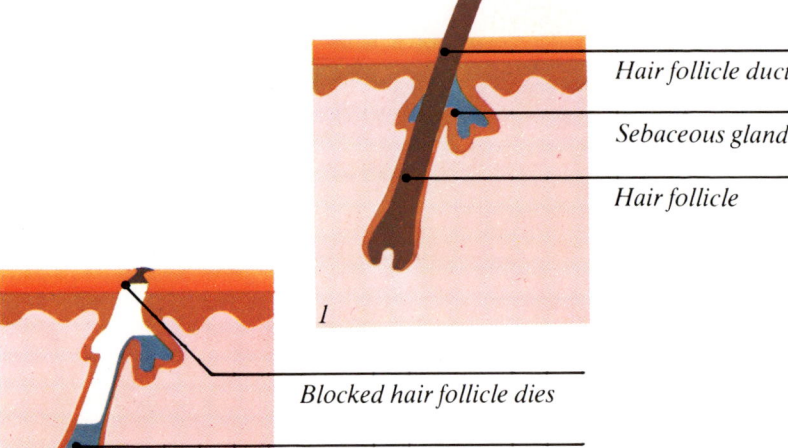

Hair follicle duct

Sebaceous gland

Hair follicle

1

Blocked hair follicle dies

Sebum

2

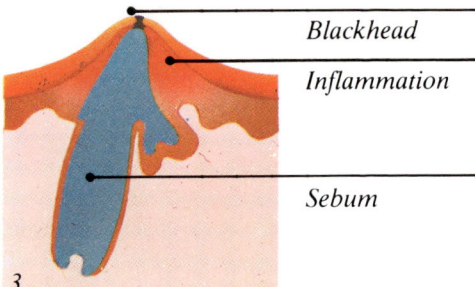

Blackhead

Inflammation

Sebum

3

Sebum normally drains along the hair follicle duct (1) and continues to be produced even if the duct becomes blocked (2). The build-up of sebum (3) leads to the formation of a blackhead.

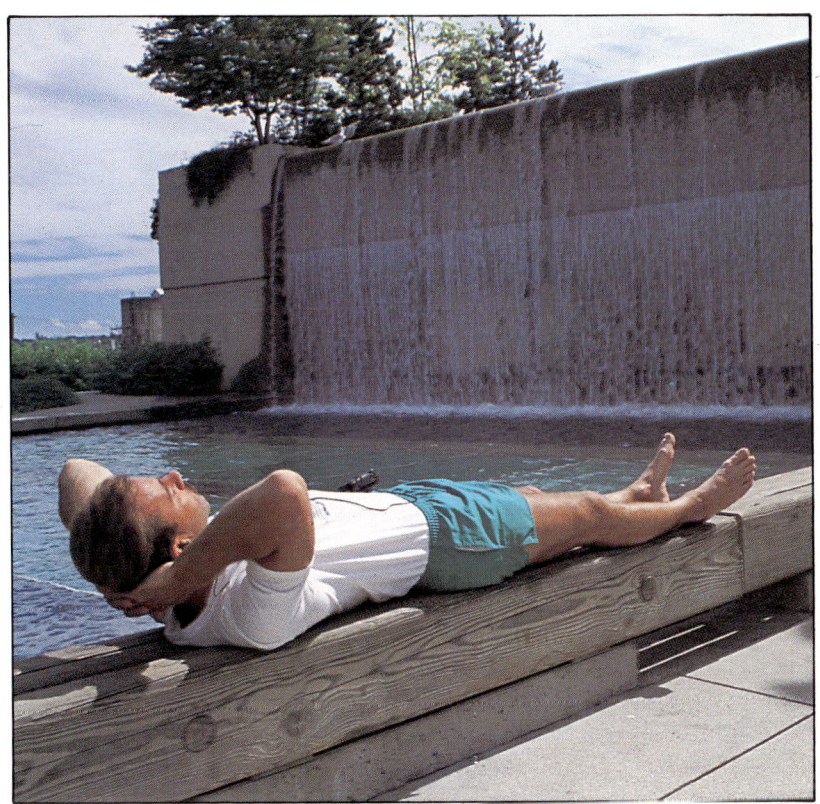

Enjoy the sun and fresh air — it's good for your skin and general health — but wear a good sunscreen.

For those who want to look youthful as long as possible, a good sunscreen is the answer.

Wrinkles on the skin cannot be avoided altogether, but taking care of the skin, moisturizing it regularly, massaging vulnerable areas, avoiding a heavy suntan, and responding positively to stress, can all help minimize wrinkles.

SKIN PROBLEMS

Acne is a skin problem that most people are at least passingly familiar with. The condition is characterized by the appearance of blackheads and pimples on the face, and occasionally on the back and chest. Acne occurs most frequently in adolescents and young adults. Scientists believe that acne is caused by a disturbance in the skin glands, which is created by certain hormone secretions.

Acne can also be an indication that the body is not eliminating toxins through the digestive system as efficiently as it could be. If constipation is also present, taking measures to treat it, such as a high-fiber diet, may help.

A severe case of acne should be treated by a dermatologist. Some foods to avoid are nuts, fats, sugar, salt, and caffeine. Foods to eat more of are green vegetables and fruits. Some dermatologists also recommend vitamins A and E, zinc, and bone meal.

Regular washing — at least once a day — with a good cleanser such as a pure castile soap, can also help treat acne. Keep the hands and hair away from the face, and above all, don't pick! Even such small details as making sure towels and pillowcases are clean can make a difference.

When the skin has been scarred because of acne, a medical treatment called dermabrasion, or skin planing, which rubs away the superficial layer of skin to the bottom of the scar, can improve the general appearance.

OTHER SKIN DISORDERS

Dermatitis is a skin rash characterized by itching, redness, and inflammation. It can be caused by irritation or sensitivities to things like wool, soaps, and oils. If an infection develops it may need to be treated with antibiotics.

Eczema is a type of dermatitis. It is an itching, oozing inflammation of the skin that appears mostly on the hands and arms. Children sometimes get eczema on the face. Eczema can be treated with skin creams prescribed by a physician.

Psoriasis is a very common type of dermatitis. It is identified by pink or red lesions surrounded by silvery scaling; they are usually found on the scalp, elbows and knees. Though there's no known cure for psoriasis, there are a number of treatments given by dermatologists that can help. Psoriasis is not contagious or life-endangering.

Sebaceous cysts are small lumps that appear under the skin, most commonly on the face, scalp, and back. They are formed in the oil-secreting, or sebaceous, glands of the skin, possibly because of poor circulation to the gland. They aren't dangerous, but if they become large they can be removed in a simple surgical procedure.

A mole is a discolored spot, usually elevated above the surface of the skin. In many cultures moles are considered beauty marks. A mole is of concern only if it begins to increase in size or change color, if it begins to bleed, or if it is irritated by clothing. Since a mole can develop into cancer, it should be examined by a physician if it shows any of these changes.

THE BRAIN

The brain is the control center of the body, the essential regulator of life. The human brain is far more complex than even the most advanced computer. It regulates all the physical aspects of life and is the seat of the mind and the emotions.

The brain is encased in the protective shell of the skull. Although the brain is very complicated, it basically consists of four major anatomical parts: the two cerebral hemispheres, the cerebellum, and the brain stem.

The *brain stem* connects the spinal cord with the rest of the brain. It controls automatic functions like breathing and the heart beat. The *cerebellum* controls muscular coordination and balance. The *cerebral hemispheres* control the senses, thought, and voluntary movement. The left cerebral hemisphere controls the right side of the body; the right cerebral hemisphere controls the left side of the body. The left side of the brain is also thought to control intuitive

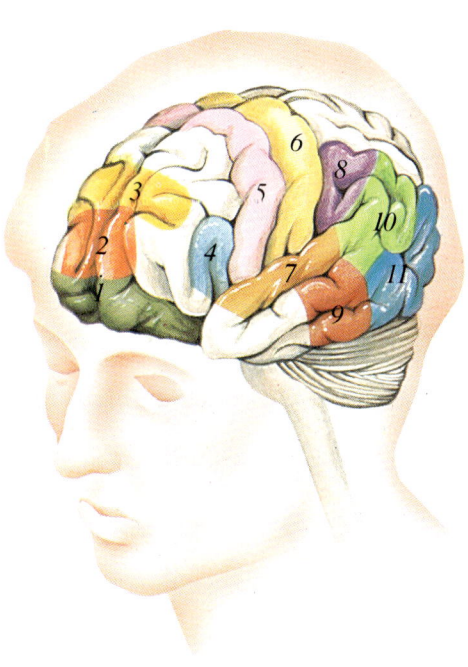

Each part of the cerebral cortex has its own function. The front lobe controls behavior (1), intellect (2) and emotion (3). The motor speech area (4) controls speech, and other sections of the motor area (5) control corresponding voluntary muscles in various parts of the body. The sensory area (6) monitors sensations from the body. The hearing center (7) registers and interprets sound. The bodily awareness center (8) integrates the information collected by the sensory area. The reading and writing centers (9,10) govern reading and writing abilities and the visual center (11) perceives and interprets images.

and creative thinking, while the right side is thought to control logical, analytical thinking.

Other important parts of the brain include the *hypothalamus,* which regulates body temperature and appetite, and the *pituitary gland,* which regulates the release of many hormones.

The four speech centers located in the cerebral hemispheres are another interesting part of the brain. These centers correspond to the four stages of growth and development of speech. The first is the auditory center, which allows a person to interpret sounds and understand language. The visual speech center is where the ability to read is developed. The motor speech center controls the muscles of the head and neck, making speech itself possible, and the written speech center gives a person the ability to read and write words.

Skull and brain injuries can vary widely in their seriousness, from a simple cut on the scalp to severe bruising of the brain and unconsciousness. However, the skull, fluids, and membranes surrounding the brain protect it very effectively.

Cuts on the scalp often appear to be much more serious than they really are because scalp wounds tend to bleed heavily. The bleeding can usually be stopped with pressure to the wound.

A concussion is a head injury resulting from a hard blow to the head that does not fracture the skull. The tissues of the brain may swell, but because they are tightly encased by the brain, the swelling cannot expand outward. Instead, it places pressure on the brain.

The most common symptom of a minor head injury is a headache starting right after the injury is received. This generally goes away in a day or two, leaving no after effects. A more serious head injury can result in unconsciousness, lasting for anywhere from just a few seconds to hours, days, or weeks (coma). Loss of consciousness for more than a few seconds can indicate a more serious injury such as a skull fracture and bleeding within the skull. Generally speaking, the longer the period of unconsciousness the more serious the injury.

Any head injury is a serious matter and should be seen by a doctor. X rays of the skull may be needed to check for a fractured skull, and the person may be admitted to the hospital for observation. Most simple concussions heal by themselves. However, a person who has received a concussion should rest and be watched carefully for a few days in case there are any complications.

The greatest danger to a person who has lost consciousness due

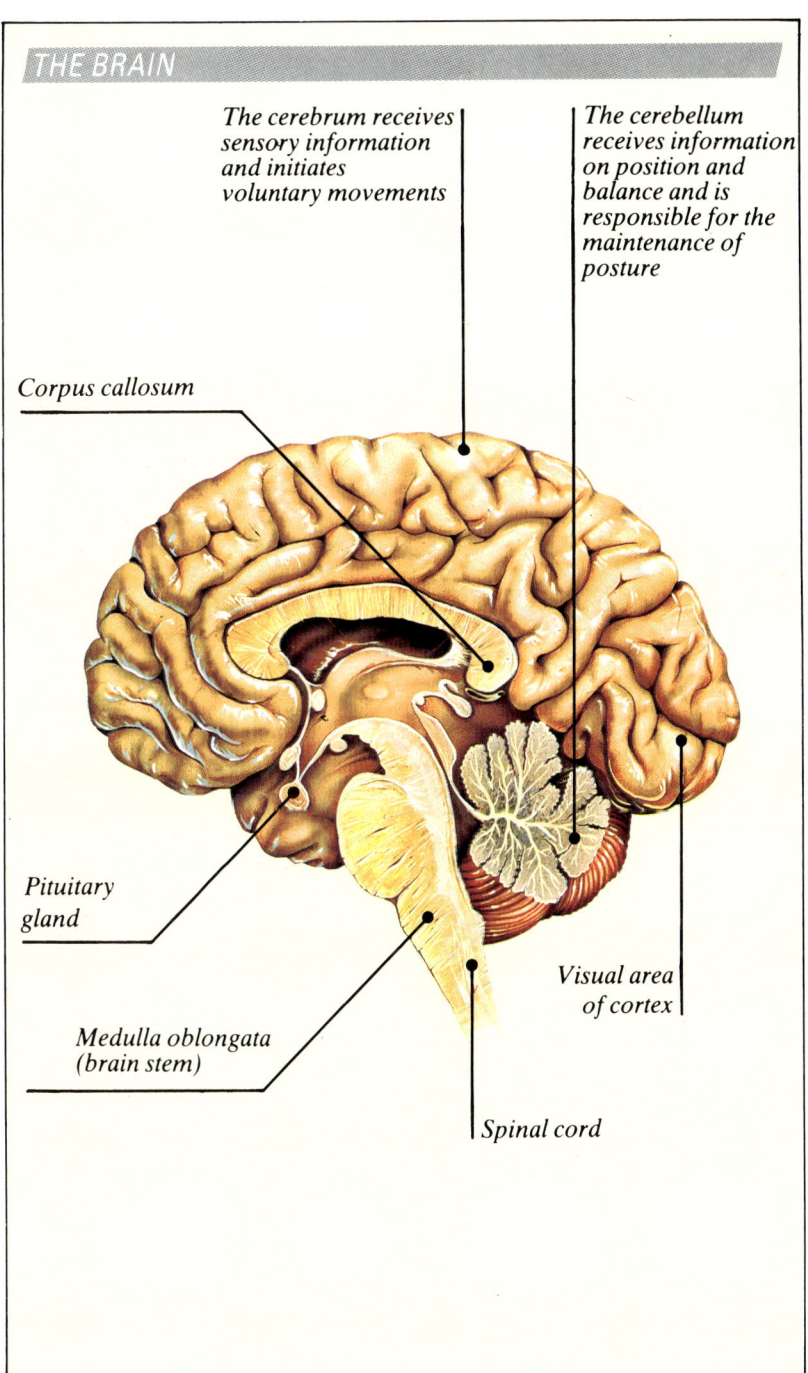

The cerebrum receives sensory information and initiates voluntary movements

The cerebellum receives information on position and balance and is responsible for the maintenance of posture

Corpus callosum

Pituitary gland

Medulla oblongata (brain stem)

Visual area of cortex

Spinal cord

to a head injury is blockage of the airway by secretions or fluids. For this reason it is important to keep an unconscious person on his or her side or sitting up slightly so that the upper body is elevated; check the airway periodically. Any bleeding should be stopped with pressure.

Bleeding within the skull may take hours, days, weeks, or even months to show up — but it is a surgical emergency whenever it happens. Symptoms of intracranial (within the skull) bleeding include increasing drowsiness, and weakness of the arms and legs on one side of the body. Symptoms that show up after a period of time may also include headache and mental confusion.

Strokes are also called cerebrovascular accidents or apoplexy, and tend to be a disorder of the elderly. They occur when the blood supply to a specific part of the brain is suddenly interrupted in some way. This can happen when a blood clot originating in the brain or carried from another part of the body closes off a blood vessel, or when a blood vessel in the brain ruptures and causes bleeding inside the brain.

Cerebral thrombosis is a condition in which an artery in the brain becomes narrower and narrower due to a thickening of its wall. Eventually the blood flow is blocked and the part of the brain normally supplied by that artery dies.

A "small" or "little" stroke (medically called a transient ischemic attack) occurs when the blood flow in a small artery of the brain is

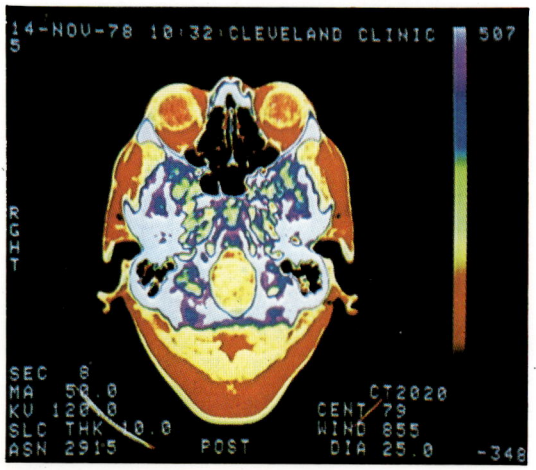

A CAT (Computerized Axial Tomography) scan involves taking a series of X-ray photographs of cross-sections of the body or head and then reconstructing them electronically. The technique is able to pinpoint which area of the brain (left) has been affected by a stroke.

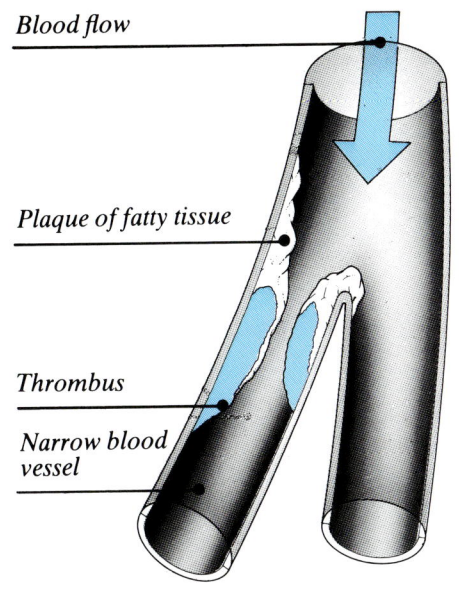

Blood flow

Plaque of fatty tissue

Thrombus

Narrow blood vessel

Thrombosis *is the formation of a clot in a blood vessel that narrows it and impedes the blood flow. If one of the vessels supplying the brain is affected, a stroke may be the result. Clots are more likely to form around atheromas, fatty deposits on the walls of blood vessels, which is why a fatty diet, high in cholesterol, has been implicated in strokes and heart disease.*

briefly interrupted. The symptoms include dizziness, headache, numbness, paralysis on one side, blurred or double vision, and temporary blindness in one eye. The symptoms may last for just a few minutes or hours, and usually go away within 24 hours, leaving little or no permanent damage. However, a "little" stroke is often a warning sign that a serious stroke could happen soon — it's estimated that nearly 75 per cent of all people who have major strokes have had the warning signs of "small" strokes. A doctor should be consulted without delay if the symptoms of a transient ischemic attack appear. Serious strokes can be prevented with proper care.

The symptoms of a serious stroke often appear suddenly and can be frightening. They can include sudden unconsciousness, numbness in an arm or leg, paralysis, confusion, blurred or double vision, inability to speak, and headache. Often the symptoms are on only one side of the body, since the damage is in one of the two cerebral hemispheres controlling that side.

Strokes require immediate medical attention.

Treatment for a stroke often involves rehabilitation to help other parts of the brain take over from the damaged areas. This can be a long process, but many stroke victims can regain a great deal of their lost abilities.

People with high blood pressure are at a greater risk of a stroke. It's a good idea to have your blood pressure checked regularly. If it is high, consult your doctor.

▶ *TENSION HEADACHES*

Tension headaches are one of the most common sources of physical discomfort in the human being, along with hunger and thirst. Every year 40 million people go to a physician complaining of severe and recurring tension headaches. A tension headache is caused when the muscles around the neck and skull contract or tighten and stay in that position, creating pressure around the skull and brain.

By far the most common cause of tension headaches is stress. When a person comes across a stressful situation in life such as overwork, personal problems, a poor physical environment, or social anxiety, the body responds. Some of the immediate physical symptoms of stress are a rapid pulse, increased blood pressure, blood flooding into the large muscle groups, increased secretion of stomach acid, shallow breathing, and secretion of adrenalin into the body.

Other, more physical, factors can also cause tension headaches. Some of those include the strain of overwork, sitting too long in one position, abnormal postures such as holding the phone between the ear and the shoulder (or anything that puts prolonged stress on the neck muscles), and sleeping on one side or with the elbow bent up below the head.

Tension headaches are usually chronic — that is, they happen regularly over a period of time. They can last from minutes to years, and tend to create a steady, generalized pain in the head and neck area. Other symptoms may include feelings of tightness in the back of the neck or forehead, soreness of the scalp, tenderness in the neck muscles, and a feeling of tightness that radiates from the neck up the back of the head and closes around the scalp in a band. There tends to be a feeling of pressure that builds and can range in intensity from minor discomfort to extreme distress.

The most effective treatments for tension headaches tend to be techniques that aim to discover and treat the cause of the headaches. These treatments may include acupuncture, counseling, chiropractic, and biofeedback (discussed later in this book). Hypnosis is often used to treat tension headaches, but has the drawback of treating only the symptom and not the cause. Non-prescription drugs such as aspirin, acetaminophen, and ibuprofen may temporarily alleviate the symptoms of a tension headache, but should not be used over a long period of time because of possible drug dependency and side-effects.

The traditional Chinese method of acupuncture may provide welcome relief for some sufferers of persistent tension headaches.

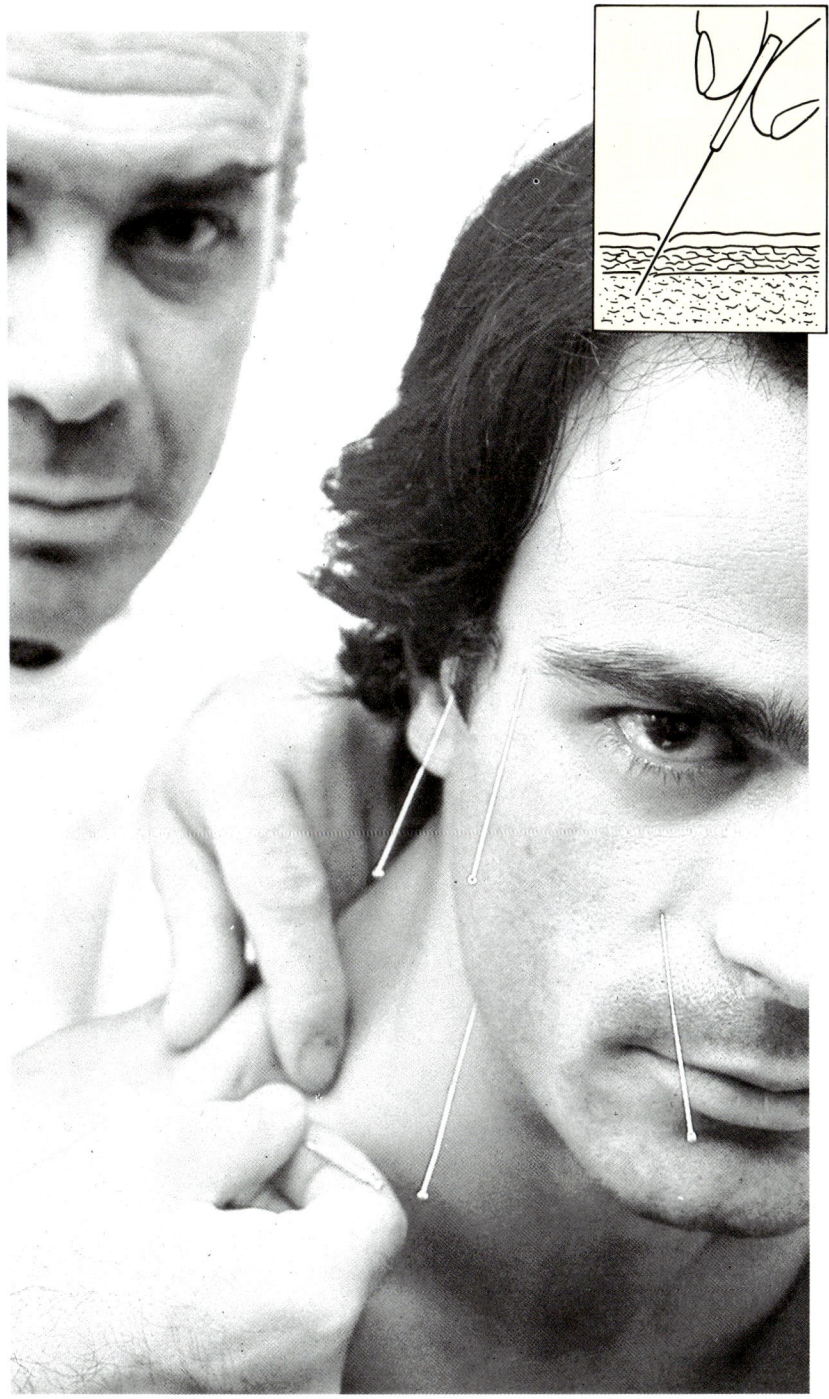

▶ *MIGRAINE HEADACHES*

Migraine or vascular headaches are caused by the dilation (expansion) of the blood vessels on the outside of the brain, causing a throbbing pain that is often excruciating. The word "migraine" is derived from the Greek word "hemicrania," which means "half a head." Many but not all migraine headaches occur on only one side of the head.

About 15 out of every 100 American adults under the age of 40 suffer from migraine headaches. The headaches may begin at any time, but usually start at puberty. An average of 75 out of every 100 migraine sufferers are women. The personality profile of migraine sufferers tends to be one of sensitive, driven, high-achievers who expect perfection from themselves and others. They tend to push themselves very hard for a period of time, such as a five-day work week, and then experience a "let-down" headache on the weekend.

Although psychological stress is thought to be the major cause of migraine headaches, there can be many other contributing factors, such as sensitivity to certain foods. People who suffer from migraines seem to have a sensitive and easily excitable chemical balance.

The symptoms of a migraine are usually very distinct from the symptoms of a tension headache. The migraine begins with what is called an "aura," which is a period from minutes to hours when the person has very cold hands and a sensation of coldness on one side of the head. This aura is created as the blood vessels in the brain

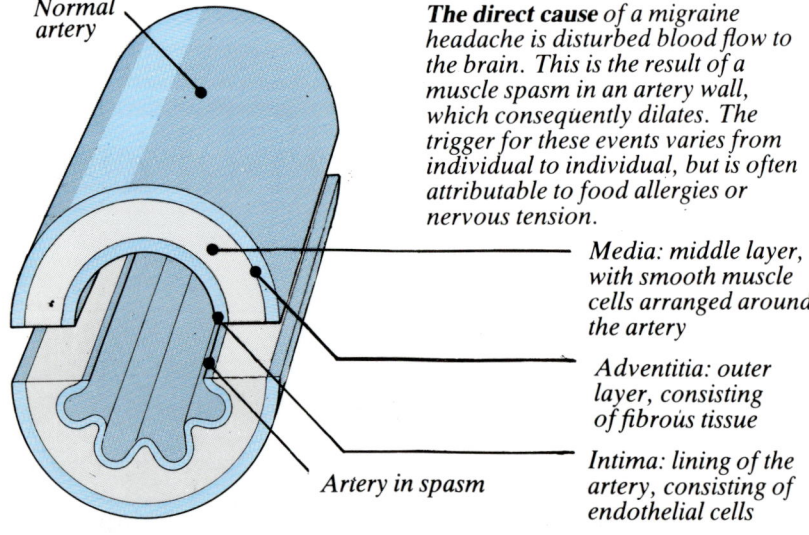

Normal artery

The direct cause of a migraine headache is disturbed blood flow to the brain. This is the result of a muscle spasm in an artery wall, which consequently dilates. The trigger for these events varies from individual to individual, but is often attributable to food allergies or nervous tension.

Media: middle layer, with smooth muscle cells arranged around the artery

Adventitia: outer layer, consisting of fibrous tissue

Intima: lining of the artery, consisting of endothelial cells

Artery in spasm

COPING WITH MIGRAINE

Although it may be relatively easy to identify a number of possible causes for migraine headaches, such as stress, anxiety and food allergies, coping with them is not always straightforward.

If you are able to detect the onset of a migraine:
- splash your face with cold water
- lie down in a darkened room and get some sleep and
- take any prescribed medications.

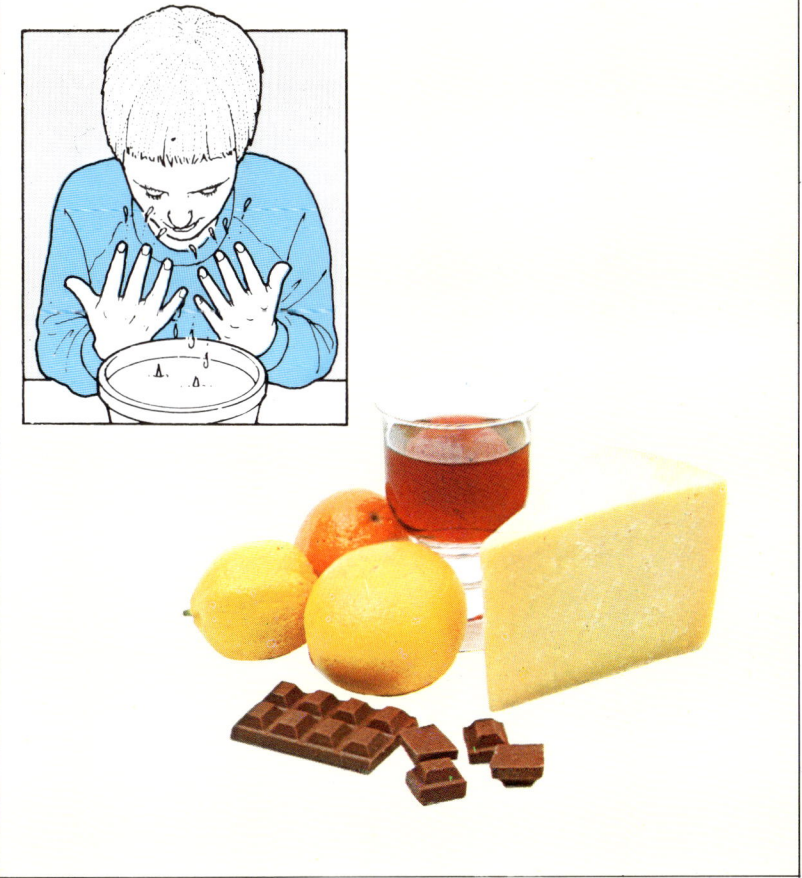

and the hands begin to narrow and go into spasm. Sometimes during the aura period people see flashing lights, and rarely, hallucinations. There may be numbness, tingling, or paralysis on one side of the body, and often a disturbance in thinking and speech. Most people also experience heavy emotional tension or negative anticipation of a stressful event before a migraine headache begins.

When the headache actually begins there is usually intense pain, caused by the flooding of fluid and inflammatory cells into the connective tissue of the brain, scalp, and facial area. Nausea may also occur.

As mentioned earlier, there are many factors that can contribute to a migraine headache. Foods that can cause the blood vessels of some sensitive people to dilate and spasm can cause a migraine. These include aged cheeses, lunch meats such as bologna and salami, pickled herring, dried fish, red wine, avocados, bananas, and canned figs. Monosodium glutamate (MSG), a food additive frequently used in processed foods, many frozen dinners, and Chinese food, is also a frequent culprit in migraines. Chocolate and peanuts are probably the two single most common foods that precipitate migraines. Other foods include liver, sour cream, foods preserved with nitrates, such as ham, bacon, and sausage, raisins, citrus fruits, olives, anchovies, and yogurt.

Beverages that can contribute to a migraine include tea, coffee, cola, champagne, bourbon, gin, and vodka. All alcoholic beverages may dilate the blood vessels. Seasonings that may contribute to a migraine include salt, Worcestershire sauce, and variations such as steak sauce, meat tenderizer, and soy sauce.

Some vitamins cause dilation of the blood vessels. Niacin (a B vitamin) is one of the most common — people who suffer from migraines should choose a vitamin with niacinamide. Too much Vitamin A can cause headaches and other side-effects as well.

About 40 out of every 100 migraine sufferers easily recognize that a few of the above substances can provoke their migraines. A good way to begin to find out which specific foods cause migraines in an individual is to eliminate all of the above listed foods from the diet over a four- to six-week period and then reintroduce them one at a time. If a specific food, beverage, or seasoning is a culprit in provoking a migraine, it will be very evident fairly quickly if the food has been avoided for at least a week and is then eaten.

Altitude changes, too much wind or sun, air pollution, a smoky or stuffy room, and high carbon monoxide levels can all contribute to migraines. Physical conditions such as hypoglycemia, premenstrual syndrome (PMS), temporal mandibular joint syndrome (TMJ) (see the section on the jaw), high blood pressure, eye strain, and dental problems may also precipitate a migraine.

There is no drug that will cure migraines. The most effective treatments include identifying food sensitivities, learning biofeedback and relaxation techniques, stress reduction, acupuncture, and exercise. When preventive measures don't work there are a few medications that may help break the pain cycle, but in general, once a migraine begins it will run its course with or without drugs. Physicians often prescribe narcotic medications such as codeine, and other drugs that may counteract the dilation of the blood vessels around the brain. Some physicians prescribe minor tranquilizers to try to help prevent attacks, but this usually only postpones the inevitable.

Drugs do not solve the problem of migraines, and actually may increase the problem because of dependency, addition, and side-effects. The key to handling migraines lies in a willingness to work carefully and closely with oneself, to be receptive to the earliest warning signs of stress, and to act upon them. If migraines function as an emotional release valve, the sufferer must be willing to find other more positive and constructive ways of relieving pressure and stress. It seems deceptively simple, yet what migraine sufferers usually need to do more than anything else is be willing to take care of themselves.

One of the most effective nondrug treatments for migraines is biofeedback, which is a system for learning to control the autonomic nervous system, which regulates functions such as body temperature and heart rate. Mastering the art of warming the cold hands that usually precede even the aura of a migraine headache can avert a headache in about 60 out of every 100 migraine sufferers. Raising the temperature of the hands can divert blood flow from the head to the hands, thus lessening the pressure and dilation of the blood vessels surrounding the brain.

Deep relaxation techniques are very effective in reducing stress, but it is important not to go into full deep relaxation during an actual migraine, because the deep relaxation state tends to dilate the blood vessels. The following exercise takes about two minutes to do, yet practicing it throughout the day can be incredibly effective in reducing stress over time, and averting migraines. This technique is adapted from the Menninger biofeedback treatment center in Topeka, Kansas.

The Two-Minute Technique is a skill or an art that can be mastered over a period of time. It's important, given the usual perfectionist profile of migraine sufferers, not to expect instantaneous success. Be patient and persistent. The Two-Minute Technique can be done any time there's a short break in the day and it's OK to allow the mind to relax — while shopping, sitting in traffic, between classes or clients, watching television, preparing a meal.

THE TWO-MINUTE TECHNIQUE

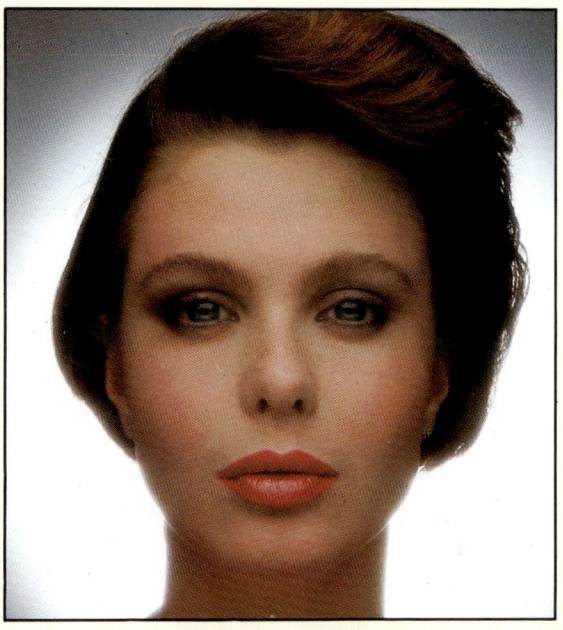

1 Become aware of your thoughts, and then switch the focus of your awareness to yourself and your breathing. Rather than trying to completely shut off the mind, just keep shifting your awareness back to yourself and your breathing if it drifts away. Take two deep breaths, inhaling slowly through the nose, and exhaling slowly through the mouth. Visualize any tensions or worries leaving with the exhaled air.

2 Beginning with the toes and working up, scan your body for any areas that may feel tense, cramped, or painful. Let go of any tension that may be present. Say to yourself, "My hands are *warm*," and warm them up now.

3 Do the following two short exercises slowly: First, gently rotate your head in circular motion once or twice, being aware of any areas where there are knots or resistance. Second, gently roll your shoulders forward and then backward a few times.

4 For just a couple of seconds, remember or picture a pleasant thought or image. This might be recalling a good time, seeing a beautiful landscape, or thinking of a loved one.

5 Take a deep breath through the nose, and exhale slowly through the mouth. Go back to whatever you were doing in a more relaxed and refreshed state.

SERIOUS HEADACHES

The vast majority of all headaches are caused by muscular contraction or tension, or by dilation of the blood vessels in the brain. Sometimes, however, headaches can be an indication of serious illnesses in the skull or brain. These are generally known as traction or inflammatory headaches.

One of the diseases that may be indicated by a severe headache is meningitis, which is an infection and inflammation of the membranes and fluids that cover and surround the brain and spinal cord. Meningitis can be caused by a number of things, including bacterial infection, an infection that spreads from the middle ear or sinuses, and viruses. Rarely, meningitis can be associated with some types of tuberculosis or syphilis.

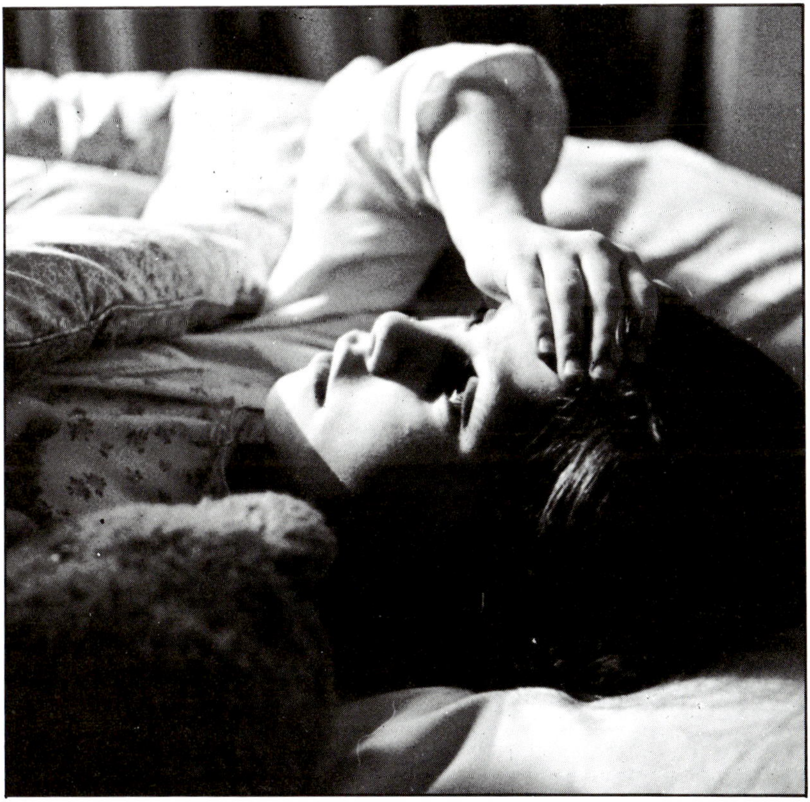

Any headache *that is accompanied by fever or which comes on very* *rapidly should be treated as serious and medical attention sought at once.*

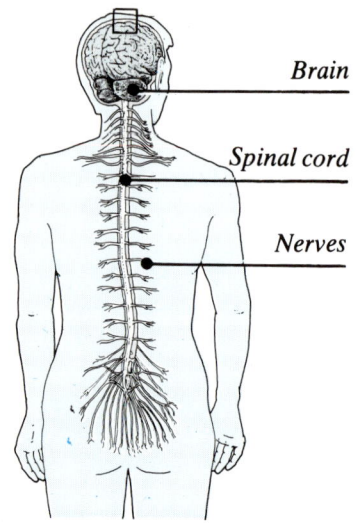

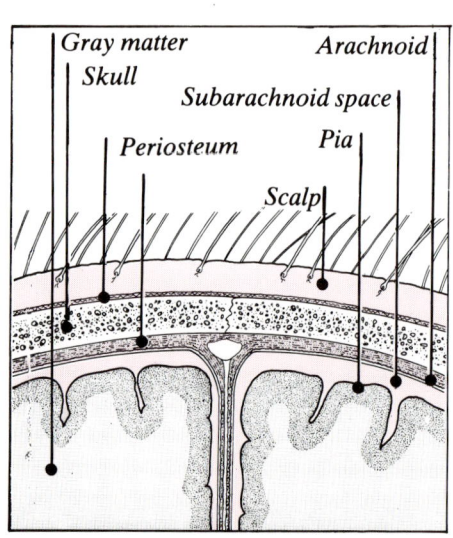

Meningitis *is an inflammation of the membranes — the meninges — that protect the brain and spinal cord.*

The symptoms of meningitis may include a sudden fever, severe headache, a stiff neck, and often a coma. The diagnosis of meningitis is made by a physician examining the spinal fluid for inflammatory cells or bacteria.

Although meningitis is a dangerous, life-threatening disease, it can be treated. Treatment varies with the cause, but is generally antibiotics or sulfa drugs.

Encephalitis is an acute inflammation of the brain. It is believed to be caused by a variety of viruses, or as a complication of measles, whooping cough, or mumps. Rarely, encephalitis occurs as a toxic reaction to severe infections such as pneumonia, typhoid fever, or any illness when there is a high fever for a long period of time. Symptoms of encephalitis may include severe headache, convulsions, fever, vomiting, paralysis, delirium, and sometimes coma. There is no specific treatment for encephalitis. While it can be fatal, the majority of patients recover completely.

If a headache comes on very suddenly, and quickly becomes severe or incapacitating (for exceptions, see the section on migraine headaches), it is important to seek medical attention right away.

Headaches may be also associated with neurological dysfunction, brain tumors, aneurysms, and other blood-vessel disorders in the brain. Those symptoms may include drowsiness, double vision, loss of vision in one eye, numbness or weakness, and difficulty with speech or coordination.

ENCEPHALITIS

A lumbar puncture
*(right) is usually
performed in the
diagnosis of
encephalitis — acute
inflammation of the
brain (below). The
condition may have a
number of causes, the
most common of which
is a viral infection.*

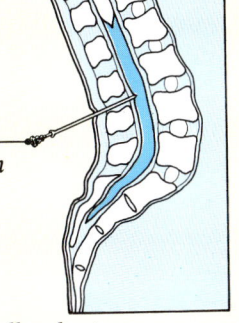

*Fluid is drawn from
the space below
the spinal cord in
the lumbar region*

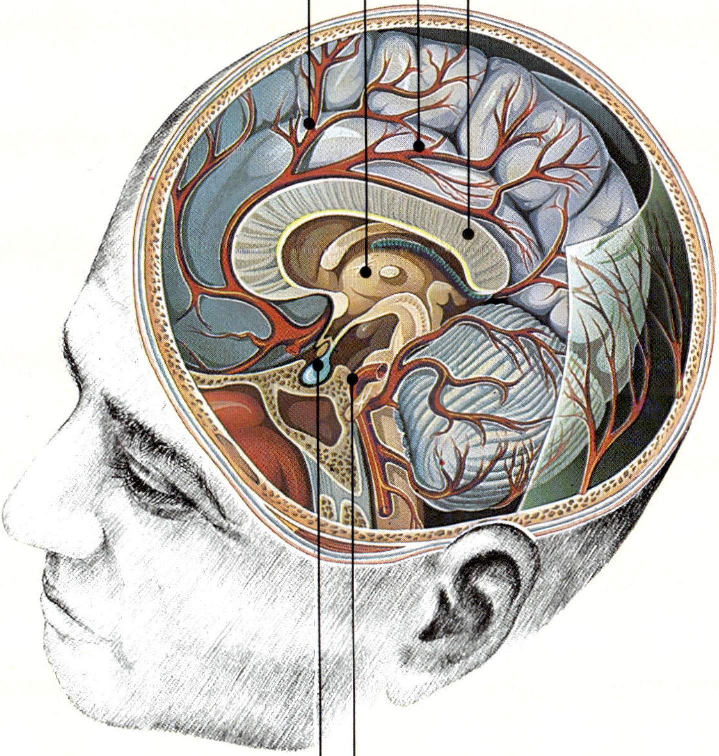

Hypothalamus

Pericallosal artery

Callosomarginal artery

Corpus callosum

Pituitary gland

Oculomotor nerve

▶ *CAUSES OF HEADACHES*

● *Hunger* can cause a headache if you have low blood sugar or hypoglycemia. These headaches generally come on between meals, or when a meal has been skipped. The treatment is to eat proteins and complex carbohydrates in small amounts frequently throughout the day.

● *Ice cream* or anything that's very cold can cause a headache if the roof of the mouth gets very cold.

● *Hot dogs* or any food preserved with sodium nitrate in it, such as bacon, sausage, lunch meats and ham, can give some people a headache.

● *MSG* (monosodium glutamate) is a flavor enhancer and food additive often used in Chinese restaurants and commonly used in many frozen, canned and processed foods. The MSG headache is usually a feeling of pressure around the temples and forehead. It can also create a feeling of pressure in the chest.

● *Too much exercise* can cause a headache if you aren't used to it. This happens because the smaller blood vessels can't keep up with all the blood being pumped through the larger blood vessels, and the blood backs up, painfully stretching the vessels.

● *Caffeine withdrawal* may cause a headache after a day or so. Caffeine shrinks the blood vessels, so when it's no longer in the system the vessels expand and cause pain. This is temporary, and usually far less painful than the long-term side-effects of a heavy caffeine habit.

● *Heavy traffic* creates thick fumes from car exhaust. The main ingredient in car exhaust is carbon monoxide, which is deadly in concentrated doses, and causes headaches in less concentrated doses. Coal, oil, and gas stoves can also give off carbon monoxide fumes.

● *PMS* (premenstrual syndrome) can cause a headache, usually along with cramps and a bloated, heavy feeling. There is speculation that PMS headaches may be caused by water retention in the brain tissues, which creates painful pressure. Vitamin B_6 may help if this is the case.

● *Going to a higher altitude,* from sea level to the mountains for example, can cause headaches, particularly when combined with one of the other possible causes listed here. It's best to avoid strenuous exercise and alcohol and drink lots of fluids for a day or so after going to a higher altitude.

● *Too much salt* in the diet is a very common cause of headaches. It's amazing how quickly the taste buds adjust to a diet with very little salt in it.

● *A stuffy room* or a smoky room can cause a headache because you're inhaling too much carbon dioxide and not enough oxygen. Sleeping with your head under the covers can have the same effect.

● *Nervous jaw movements* such as rocking, clenching, and grinding the jaws and teeth can cause headaches. Handling stress before it gets to the jaw is the best treatment.

● *Poor posture* can put a strain on the neck and shoulder muscles, which then radiates up into the skull and causes a headache. Sitting in front of a typewriter all day, slumping, reading in bed with your head propped forward, and sleeping with too many pillows can all create a headache.

● *Overexposure to the sun* can cause the body to become dehydrated, which can cause a headache. A more serious form of this is sunstroke. Wear sunscreen, a hat, and loose, cool clothes in you need to be in the sun for a long time.

● *Sleeping too much,* too little, or at odd hours, can cause a headache.

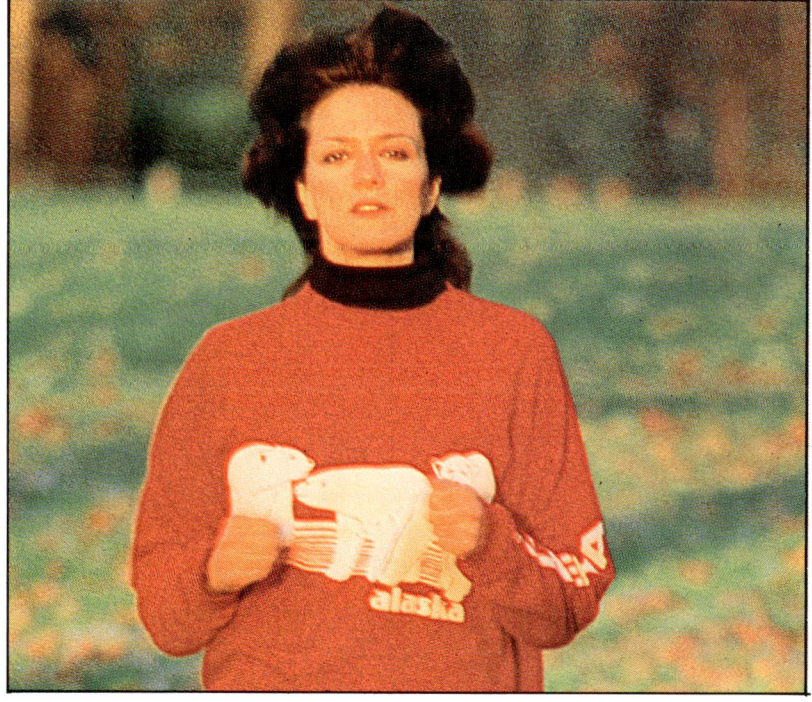

Unaccustomed exercise *may bring on a headache because small blood vessels can't cope with the rate at which blood is being pumped through larger vessels. The blood backs up and stretches the vessels to cause pain.*

DEALING WITH PAIN

How we feel pain and what we can do about it has been the subject of a great deal of scientific research recently. Traditionally, pain was thought to be a simple bodily response to a stimulus, so that the amount or degree of pain experienced was directly related to the source of the pain. Thus, the medical approach to pain was to get rid of the source of the pain as quickly as possible often with drugs or surgery. Drugs are certainly important in pain control, but they only relieve symptoms and can cause serious side-effects, including addition. Surgery is now rarely recommended for the relief of chronic pain.

What researchers have discovered in the past few years is that while pain is, of course, related to the stimulus, individual reactions to it are also a major factor in the perception of pain. Furthermore, every individual reacts to pain in a unique way. Studies indicate that people exposed to identical painful stimuli react with a wide variety of responses, and even the same person's reaction to the same painful stimulus can vary greatly under different conditions. What these studies conclude is that psychological factors play a large part in the perception of pain. And if these factors can increase pain, they can also reduce it.

This is known as the "gate theory." It is believed that the nerves in the brain responsible for receiving and transmitting pain messages can alter the individual's perception of pain by opening and closing — just like a gate. The theory suggests that the perception of pain can be influenced effectively through positive thoughts and attitudes.

It is now thought that there are many natural ways to stimulate the release of those chemicals in the brain that relieve pain and create a sense of well-being. These chemicals, called endorphin, serotonin, and norepinephrine, are thought to work together to relieve pain and move it into what might be called a state of discomfort.

The endorphins are located in the pituitary gland, the temporal lobe of the brain, in the digestive system, and in the adrenal gland. They have been found to work the same way morphine does to relieve pain. The temporal lobe of the brain is related to feeling, and contains large amounts of endorphins.

It has been recently discovered that endorphins are released in fairly large quantities during strenuous exercise, accounting for the feeling of well-being popularly known as "runner's high." It is also possible that endorphins may be released as a result of deep relaxation, positive visualization, laughing, and other positive experiences that elicit a sense of well-being.

Pain is sensation extended beyond a level that is comfortable. The nervous system's response to stimuli depends, among other things, on the sense of touch — whether an object is rough or smooth, for example, or wet or cold.

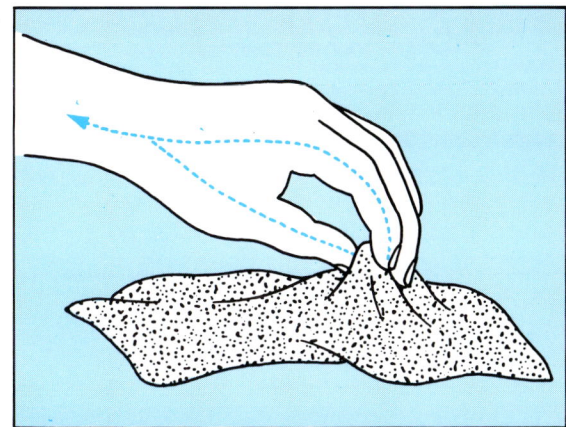

Sensation is also involved in relaying information about whether a given stimuli is too hot and likely to cause burning.

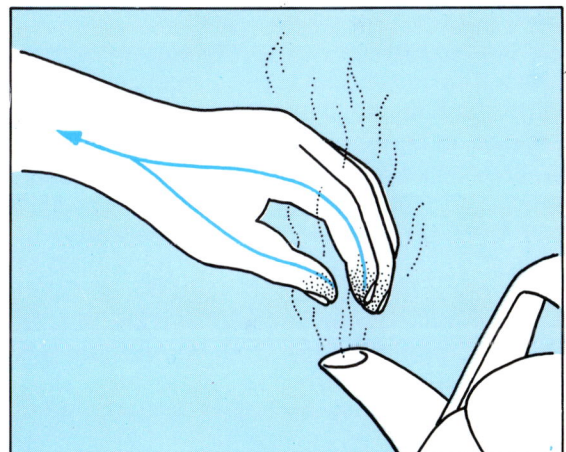

The perception of pain forms part of the body's defense mechanism, giving warning of situations or events that may cause physical injury or be hazardous to health.

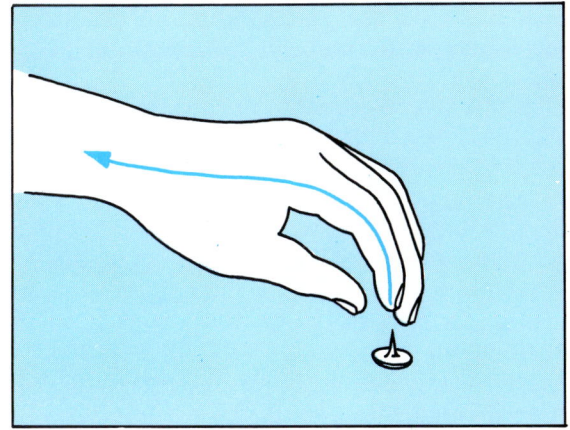

▶ *ACUPUNCTURE*

Acupuncture is one of the most ancient forms of healing on the earth. The Chinese have been practicing acupuncture for at least 5,000 years — it is one of the most vital elements of their sophisticated traditional medicine.

Acupuncture treatments are usually carried out by inserting needles into very specific points on the body. The Chinese practitioner of medicine treats the patient as a whole entity consisting of the mind, emotions, and body; the practitioner looks for the cause of an illness rather than treating a symptom.

One of the fundamentals of Chinese medicine is the concept of the polarities or opposites of yin and yang, which are present in all of life. These represent polarities such as hot–cold, love–hate, dark–light, active–passive, hard–soft, odd–even, heavy–light, contraction–expansion, sour–sweet, wet–dry, strong–weak, sun–moon, left–right, high–low, heaven–earth, masculine–feminine. Other fundamental concepts are the Ch'i Energy, which is the vital force in all of life, and the Tao, which is the path or the rhythm on or in which one may sustain the pure Ch'i energy. The Tao is a process of maintaining and attuning to a balance between the yin and yang. In yin and yang the opposites do not clash; they are constantly changing and transforming from one to the other.

It's not difficult to apply these beautiful and poetic concepts to balance and harmony in the body. The purpose of acupuncture is to assist the patient in restoring equilibrium to whatever has become imbalanced. According to the theory, the Ch'i circulates along specific channels, or meridians, in the body; to maintain a healthy body, the Ch'i must circulate freely in the proper strength and quality. Acupuncture controls the Ch'i energy at special points located on the meridians. Through the meridians run throughout the body, inside and out, acupuncture points are mostly on the surface of the body.

Acupuncture gained increased respectability in the West when it was discovered that it can cause the release of endorphins and enkephalins, natural substances in the body that create a sense of well-being and reduce pain in much the same way that morphine does. Many people experience a dreamy or euphoric state during acupuncture treatments, which may be due to the release of these substances. It may also be the release of endorphins and enkephalins that is responsible for the analgesic (pain-relieving) effects of acupuncture. Acupuncture treatments can be immediately effective in pain relief, and also may help with long-term chronic pain. This phenomenon may also provide a rational explanation for the fact that major surgery has been safely performed without the use of anesthesia, and with the patient fully conscious, using acupuncture.

The first part of an acupuncture treatment is diagnosis. The appearance of the tongue is an important diagnostic tool. The Chinese doctor is trained to ask about the symptoms, to listen to the sound of the voice and what is said, to observe facial expressions, signs and symptoms, posture, color of the skin, and so forth, and finally to feel the skin, its temperature and texture, and to feel the pulse.

It is the Chinese doctor's ability to make a sophisticated and detailed diagnosis of a patient through nothing but the pulse that has probably most impressed Western doctors. The Chinese doctor uses three fingers on each wrist to feel the pulse, giving a total of six pulses, which are each felt at three different degrees of pressure: superficial, medium, and deep. At least 28 categories of pulse can be described, such as length, width, rhythm, rate, and overall quality. Learning to read the pulses is an art that requires many years of training and experience.

In a traditional acupuncture session, from five to 15 points are stimulated by inserting needles, which are usually left in place for about 20 minutes. The needles may be manipulated every few minutes by rotating them back and forth by lifting them in and out. Most people report that acupuncture is painful in a certain sense of the word. There may be some pain when the needle is inserted (acupuncture rarely causes bleeding) and later possibly a dull, aching sensation in the general area. However, the overall sensation of an acupuncture session is usually very pleasant.

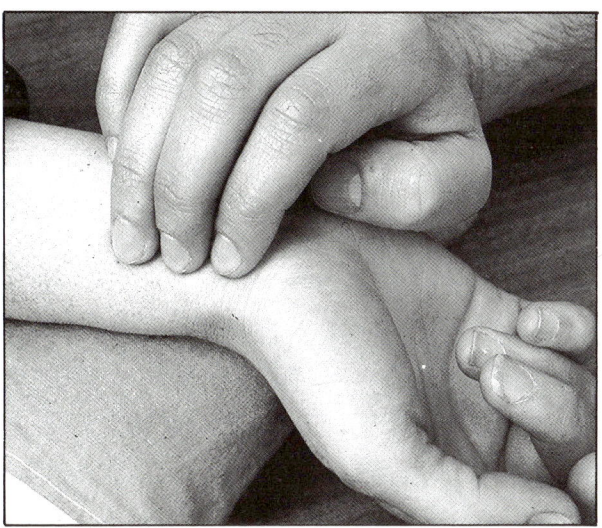

Rather than taking just one pulse, the acupuncturist measures three pulses in each wrist. Subtle variations in the quality of each are said to give clear indications of which organs are disordered and the nature and severity of the patient's condition.

▶ *HYPNOSIS*

Hypnosis is a very ancient form of inducing a state of relaxation and exerting control over the consciousness of another person. Its first use and study in the Western countries was done by Franz Mesmer, an eighteenth-century physician who lived in Paris. The term to "mesmerize," or hypnotize, was coined for Mesmer.

Hypnosis can induce a state of deep relaxation. It is better known for the fact that the hypnotist can give direct suggestions which the patient may follow without even being aware that they have been given. Though there is still no scientific or logical explanation for how hypnosis works, it is a fairly commonly accepted form of treatment for any number of ailments. It is used by doctors, dentists, and therapists. Hypnosis most likely produces an altered state of consciousness, and seems to work especially well with children.

A wide variety of disorders are treated with hypnosis. One of the most common uses is suppressing pain. This may be as basic as using hypnosis in the dentist's chair or as profound as using it in place of anesthetics during surgery. It is used successfully to help people lose weight and quit smoking. Most hypnotherapy, as it is called, focuses on relieving symptoms such as headaches, insomina, anxiety, and skin disorders. Some health-care specialists question the wisdom of removing symptoms without addressing the underlying cause, which may be physical, emotion, or mental. Sometimes the symptoms may disappear completely, but sometimes other symptoms may take their place — it all depends upon the individual.

It is very important to choose a hypnotherapist on the basis of reliable recommendations, and to choose one whom you trust. Putting your consciousness in the control of another person to treat an illness does involve some risk.

SELF-HYPNOSIS

Self-hypnosis is a form of positive visualization. If done properly it can be extremely effective in treating a wide variety of problems, from weight control to pain. Usually self-hypnosis involves what is called a guided meditation, which may be narrated or put on a cassette tape. Self-hypnosis usually has the most benefit if used at least once a day for at least 32 days.

Guided meditation and positive visualization are becoming a commonly accepted treatment for cancer patients. Bringing a positive focus to the disease can effect dramatic changes in both the patient's psychological outlook and the health of his or her body.

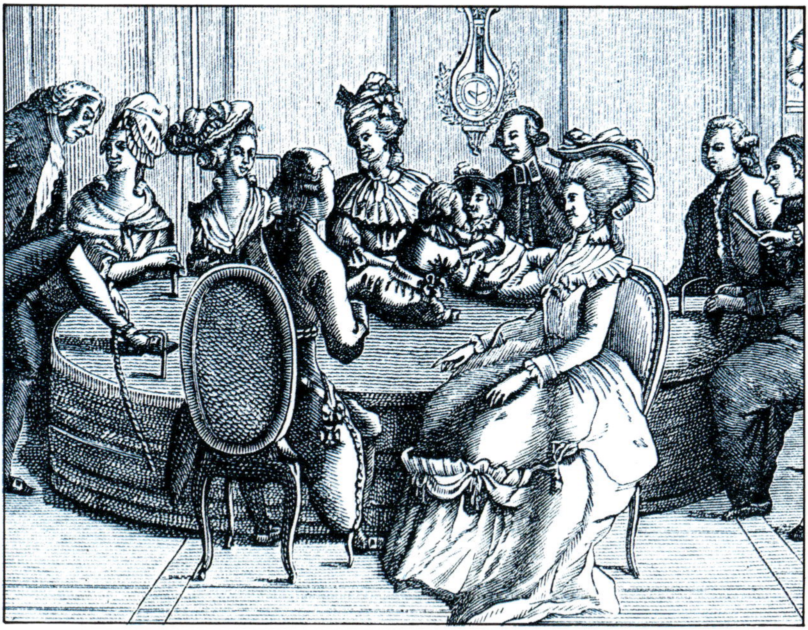

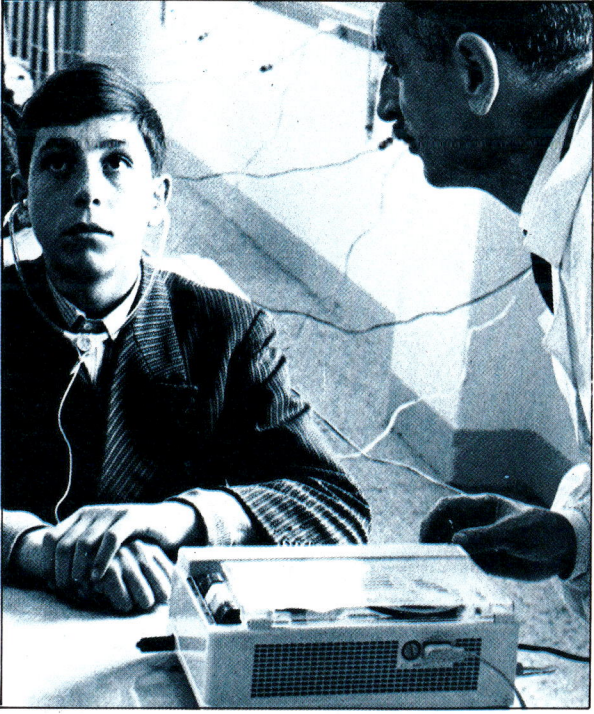

An early form of hypnotism was developed by the eighteenth-century physician Friedrich Anton Mesmer, who was able to induce a trance-like state in his subjects *(above)* through a technique he called "animal magnetism." **When hypnotized** *(left)*, a person is likely to be more receptive than normal, and for this reason hypnotism is sometimes used as an aid to learning.

▶ *BIOFEEDBACK*

Biofeedback is a recently developed technique for using the mind to help regulate, balance, and relax the body and the emotions. It was once thought that internal body states such as temperature and blood pressure were completely involuntary and not within the reach of our conscious control. Now we know that the conscious mind is capable of controlling most bodily functions to very subtle levels.

Most of us use some form of feedback in our lives every day: stepping on a scale gives feedback about weight; the speedometer of a car gives feedback about how the accelerator or brake is being used; and a thermometer gives feedback about the temperature of the body.

Mind-over-body biofeedback involves watching sensitive machines (some of which can be elegantly simple and inexpensive) that give you information about how your body is functioning. In biofeedback training you use this information to learn to monitor and control a body process. Learning the techniques doesn't take any special sensitivity or intelligence — it simply takes a little bit of instruction and practice. Consequently almost anyone can learn to regulate the pulse rate, body temperature, or muscle tension simply, easily and effectively.

Some of the more common ailments that may respond well to biofeedback are high blood pressure, migraine and tension headaches, asthma, back and neck tension and pain, stress-related tension, colitis, cerebral palsy, epilepsy, some kinds of arthritis and heart problems, and drug and alcohol withdrawal. Biofeedback has become an almost standard treatment for relieving headache pain. Stroke and paralysis victims have used biofeedback to regain muscle control by learning to regulate muscle control through other senses. People who use biofeedback often report relief of physical symptoms, and a sense of psychological well-being, as they learn to master their bodily responses.

On most biofeedback machines, sensors are attached to the skin to monitor the temperature or electrical charge; a visual or auditory signal, such as a light or buzzer, signals changes in the response. The trainer gives instructions on how to work with the signals. The technique can be as simple as imagining that you are holding your hands over a campfire to warm them up. Although receiving instruction from somebody trained in biofeedback, on a very sensitive machine, is ideal, a biofeedback machine can be as simple as holding an inexpensive thermometer in the hand and observing the mercury as it rises and falls.

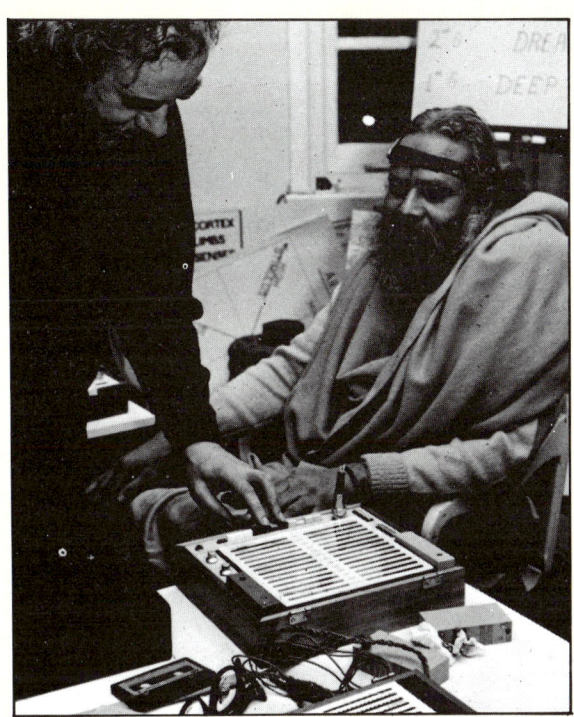

Experiments have been conducted with biofeedback apparatus (left) to investigate how certain Indian adepts are able to exert voluntary control over various body functions.
Blood pressure is measured by wrapping an inflated cuff round the arm to stop the blood flow, then deflating it gradually until the blood starts to flow again. This can be detected by feeling the pulse (below).

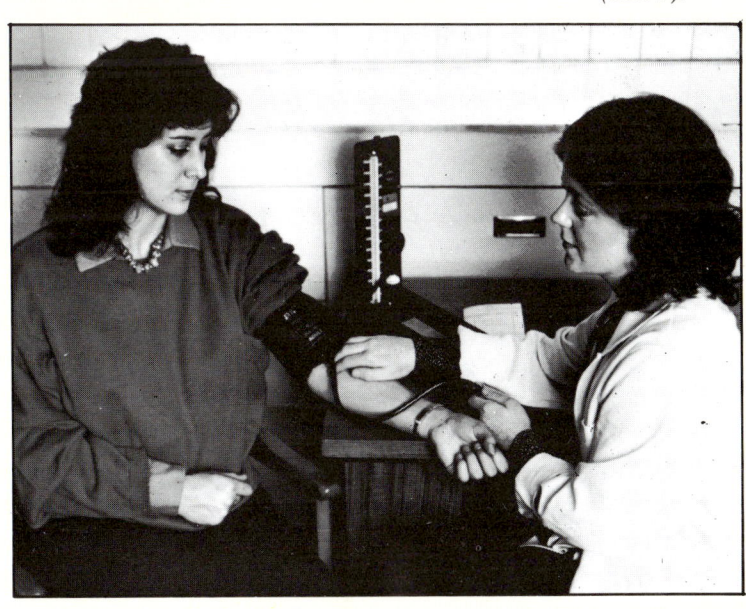

81

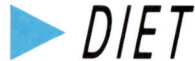 # *DIET*

The food we eat is an important part of our overall health and well-being. Maintaining a healthy diet can help prevent disease and lead to better performance in all aspects of life, including exercise, work, and personal relationships. Keeping the body at a healthy weight can improve your physical health and self-esteem. Ironically, the typical Western diet, heavy in sugar, animal fat, refined and processed foods, additives, preservatives and insecticides, is a major cause of disease. For most of the world, simply being able to eat regularly is considered a healthy diet. In the industrialized nations of the world, overeating is a far greater threat to health than not getting enough food.

Since the 1960s there has been a gradual trend toward a diet that emphasizes more so-called natural foods. This trend was spurred when people began to realize how many of the nutrients in their food were being processed out through canning, freezing, cooking, and refining. Without the added vitamins, a slice of white bread has virtually no nutritional value, and may actually create more overall harm than good in the digestive system. Canned foods lose most of their nutritional content during processing. Frozen foods are better, but there is no substitute for whole, fresh foods.

In addition to losing nutritional value, most fruits, grains, and vegetables are contaminated with herbicides and insecticides, many of which have never been tested for safety. Much of the soil that grains and vegetables are grown in is overused and depleted of minerals, which means that whatever is grown in it is also depleted of minerals. Most seafood is at least mildly contaminated by ocean pollution created by decades of using the oceans as a waste-disposal system. Our cattle, pigs, and chickens are pumped full of anti-biotics and growth stimulants that may or may not be present in the flesh when it's eaten by consumers. Increasing evidence is pointing to these kinds of food contamination as a major contributing factor to disease.

Another contributing dietary factor to disease is the fact that most of the bulk, or fiber, has been refined and processed out of Western diets. Fiber in the diet aids the digestive system in passing food through, and has a cleansing effect on the digestive tract. Lack of fiber can create infection and disease in the digestive tract, making it much more difficult for the digestive system to absorb nutrients. Fiber is found in fresh fruit and vegetables, and whole grains, including rice.

Many people in Western, industrial societies suffer from chronic, low-grade symptoms of poor digestion without even knowing it.

Constant gas, bloating, stomach cramps, constipation, diarrhea and fatigue, are an all-too-common part of everyday life. What most people with chronic, diet-related digestive problems don't realize is that their energy and performance levels are also much lower than they might be.

Cholesterol is thought to be another major dietary factor in disease. It is a substance found only in animal products, including meat, cheese, butter, eggs, and milk. Too much cholesterol in the diet, usually combined with not enough exercise, causes fatty deposits to build up inside artery walls, which leads to heart disease. One of the worse high-fat offenders is fast food. A typical fast-food hamburger with all the fixings contains more than 12 tablespoons of fat. Although the human diet doesn't require a lot of fat, it is important, and can be found in nuts, grains, and in many vegetables such as corn and soybeans.

Maintaining a healthy diet is as simple as following these guidelines:

● Make fresh fruits and vegetables the mainstay of the diet. There are many, many ways to prepare easy, tasty vegetable dishes.

● Eat raw, uncooked, and unprocessed fruits and vegetables whenever possible. Many nutrients can be lost through cooking, particularly boiling. Steam rather than boil food whenever possible.

● Avoid refined sugar whenever possible. Eat fruits, which contain a form of sugar, to satisfy a sweet tooth.

● Cut down on salt.

● Avoid refined white flour. Make the switch to whole grains.

● Eat more fiber in the form of whole grains. There are also many high-fiber cereals on the market now.

● Reduce the amount of animal fat in the diet by cutting down on red meat and dairy products.

● Avoid foods that are canned, bottled, processed, and frozen. Their vitamin and mineral content is generally low, and they usually contain chemicals and additives. Many condiments such as mustard, ketchup, mayonnaise, pickles, and steak sauce also contain sodium, chemicals and additives.

● Drink plenty of fluids. From four to six glasses of water a day will help flush toxins and waste from the body. Herbal teas, hot or iced, such as camomile, peppermint, and hibiscus are safe, delicious, and can actually have beneficial effects.

▶ *STRESS*

Stress is very much a disease of the twentieth century. As popularly used, the word "stress" refers to feelings of pressure, excitement, nervousness, fatigue, or exhaustion that may be caused by demands from both within and without. It's important to realize that we create stress within ourselves as much as or more than any factor in the outside world causes it.

Anything that happens in our inner or outer world that demands a change, an adjustment, or a response of some kind, whether physical, mental, or emotional, is called a "stressor." However, the body responds physically to these demands, with great sensitivity, whether or not the demand itself is physical.

This bodily response is a "fight or flight" mechanism — a response that was appropriate for our cave-dwelling and hunting ancestors, whose lives would be in danger if their body wasn't prepared to either fight or run away. We are rarely in those kinds of life-threatening situations now, but our bodies react the same way to a perceived threat. Instead of saber-toothed tigers, modern-day threats could be a late paycheck, a traffic jam, or a disagreement with a loved one.

When we perceive a stressor in our environment, our body reacts and responds quickly and efficiently. These responses can include rapid heart rate or pulse, rapid, shallow breathing, perspiration and sweaty palms, muscles tightening, increased blood-sugar level which gives us immediate energy, and constriction of the blood vessels. The stomach tightens and releases acid, adrenalin, which can give a sense of heightened concentration and attention, is released into the bloodstream, and we may experience emotional edginess or emotional changes such as rage, fear, anger, or anxiety.

To add to the problem of all these physical reactions with "no place to go," we also have a cultural taboo that says it is not OK to express anger when we feel it, and it is not OK to express our emotional needs in general. So we bottle it up inside, thus creating tremendous internal pressure, both physically and emotionally.

Scientific studies show that it is healthier to express anger. Bottling anger up can contribute to serious illnesses — heart attacks, strokes, ulcers, high blood pressure, and most commonly, tension or migraine headaches.

Extreme stress may create extreme anxiety, phobias, paranoia, depression, aggression, confused thinking, and other signs of psychological disturbance. Stress is also being implicated in diseases of the immune system and some types of cancer.

Some of the most common stressors include:

● The pressure of overwork, too much work, and deadlines.
● Demands from many areas in a person's life, such as the working mother and wife who is responding to demands from her workplace, children, husband, and other family members.
● Change in lifestyle, or an important event such as a birth, death, marriage, divorce, changing jobs, and moving.
● Upsets, conflicts and disagreements with others, particularly loved ones.
● Difficulty or frustration in meeting personal needs such as loss of income, lack of relationship, even hunger and thirst.
● The loss of something or someone we care for or depend on. This might be a relationship, a pet, a job, a home.
● Social anxiety, which usually means a perceived threat to our personal well-being or self-esteem.

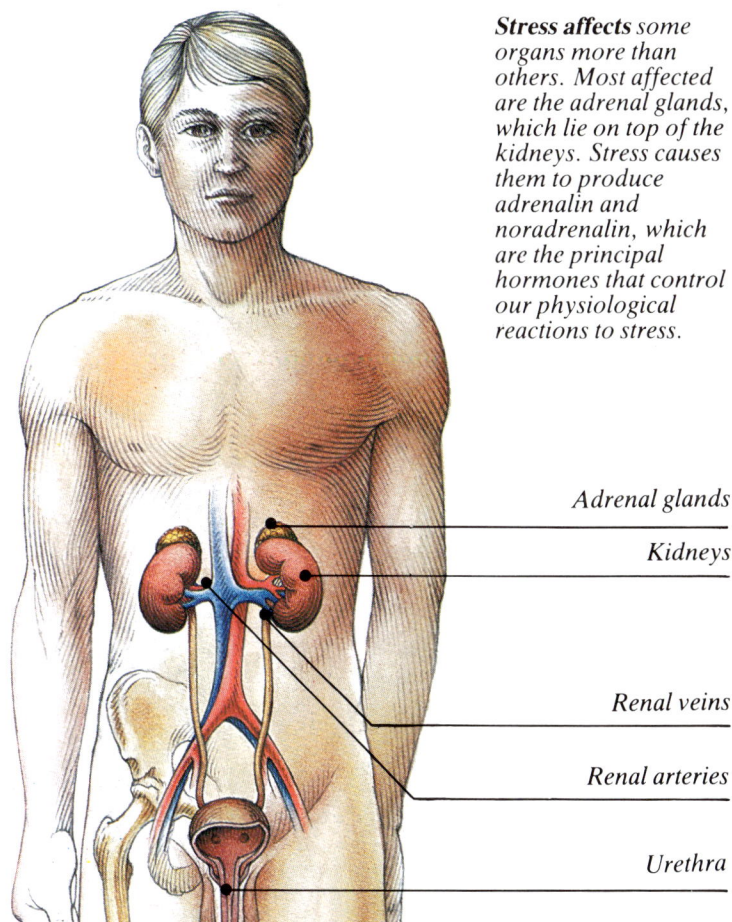

Stress affects some organs more than others. Most affected are the adrenal glands, which lie on top of the kidneys. Stress causes them to produce adrenalin and noradrenalin, which are the principal hormones that control our physiological reactions to stress.

Adrenal glands

Kidneys

Renal veins

Renal arteries

Urethra

COPING WITH STRESS

A state of tension or anxiety is what we feel when we experience stress and at the same time believe there's no way out of it. People often describe this as a feeling of being trapped, which creates an intolerable sense of pressure. There are many, many ways, both positive and negative, of coping with stress and the resulting tension. Some of the most common positive forms of coping with tension and relieving it are exercise, relaxation, meditation, discussing problems with a friend or counselor, hobbies, and diversions such as movies. Coping can be as simple as taking ten minutes to watch a sunset, or eating a hot, nourishing meal. Most people are also familiar with methods of coping that tend to have short- or long-term negative results — overeating, alcohol abuse, smoking, drug use, withdrawal, habitual anger and blaming, and denying.

Psychological factors are equally important in coping with stress. It is important to know and be aware that a stressful response to situations that are aggravating can be changed. We get caught up in the habits and routines of our lives and forget that we have choices. Creating a sense of objectivity by stepping out of the routine, even for a moment, can dramatically change your outlook on life. Cultivating a sense of responsibility for all aspects of life can be risky for many people, but is ultimately a very empowering position. Placing responsibility on someone or something else, from society, to a boss, or to a traffic jam, puts personal power outside oneself. Taking personal power and control over your life means, above all, taking full responsibility.

Another key to coping with stress is being aware of which demands in life are creating a stressful response, and then either changing the situation or the response. Most people are in the middle of a panic, fear, or anxiety response before they're even aware of it. Simply having the intention to become aware of a stressful response is a very effective first step in handling stress.

It's sometimes difficult for people to pinpoint exactly what is causing stress or to realize just how stressful some life events can be. This chart can help you determine how much stress your life contains. If you have recently experienced any of the possible events listed here, write down the number of points assigned to each. Add up the numbers. If the total is 150 or more, you are experiencing a lot of stress.

STRESS FACTORS

	Life Event	Value
1	Death of a spouse	100
2	Divorce	73
3	Marital separation	65
4	Jail term	63
5	Death of a close family member	63
6	Personal injury or illness	53
7	Marriage	50
8	Losing job	47
9	Marital reconciliation	45
10	Retirement	45
11	Change in health of a family member	44
12	Pregnancy	40
13	Sex difficulties	39
14	Addition of a new family member	39
15	Business readjustment	39
16	Change in financial state	38
17	Death of a close friend	37
18	Change to different line of work	36
19	Change in number of arguments with spouse	35
20	Mortgage over $10,000	31
21	Foreclosure of mortgage or loan	30
22	Change in responsibilities at work	29
23	Son or daughter leaving home	29
24	Trouble with in-laws	29
25	Outstanding personal achievement	28
26	Spouse begins or stops work	26
27	Begin or end school	26
28	Change in living conditions	25
29	Revision of personal habits	24
30	Trouble with boss	23
31	Change in work hours or conditions	20
32	Change in residence	20
33	Change in schools	20
34	Change in recreation	19
35	Change in church activities	19
36	Change in social activities	18
37	Mortgage or loan less than $10,000	17
38	Change in sleeping habits	16
39	Change in number of family get-togethers	15
40	Change in eating habits	15
41	Vacation	13
42	Christmas	12
43	Minor violations of the law	11

Total Points

▶ *ATTITUDE*

The way we choose to perceive the world and ourselves in it is a major factor in how well we function in the world. What we tell ourselves is what we create around us. If we're constantly giving ourselves negative messages, criticizing ourselves and others, blaming ourselves and others, we're likely to have negative experiences. On the other hand, if we give ourselves positive messages, understanding, praise, patience, and nurturing, we're likely to have positive experiences.

The thoughts we choose to focus upon have tremendous power in our lives. The words we choose to speak to ourselves can affect our outlook on life, our energy level, our productivity, and our relationships with others.

For example, take a salesperson in a retail store. A potential customer comes in the door and the salesperson is saying to herself: "Oh darn, here comes another person who probably doesn't want to buy anything. She's just going to waste my time, and besides my head hurts, my feet ache, and I don't like her haircut." That attitude is going to be picked up, on some level, by the potential customer, who will probably exit quickly without buying anything. Let's say the salesperson is saying this within herself: "Oh good, here comes a potential customer. Even if she doesn't buy anything we might have an interesting conversation — I might even make a new friend. Having people in the store makes the day pass quickly." Even if the customer doesn't buy anything on this visit, she will remember the friendly attitude of the salesperson and be more likely to return, and the salesperson will feel happier. Making the switch from negative to positive self talk is a choice.

Changing negative self talk to positive self talk is a matter of changing a habit pattern. One of the most fun and easy ways to do this is to create affirmations. These are positive statements, stated in the present tense. For example, someone preparing to give a presentation in front of a group, but who feels unsure of expressing herself clearly might create this affirmation: "I am expressing myself clearly and confidently." (Notice the use of "I am" rather than "I will." Using "I will" always puts the desired state into the future. "I am" makes it present at the moment.) Saying this affirmation out loud or inside whenever doubt about the presentation comes up can create a very real sense of clarity and confidence.

Affirmations are meant to be used regularly — sometimes the problem is remembering to use them.

Some people like to begin and end their day with affirmations and positive visualizations of how they would like the day to be.

POSITIVE AFFIRMATIONS

Below are examples of some positive affirmations. Affirmations are very individual, so use them if they fit, or take them only as examples and then create your own. Keep the following guidelines in mind: State everything positively. Avoid the use of words like, not, don't, no, never, won't, and so on. Keep it in the present, so that you really get the message that you want this positive state to be present right now. Keep it general — you never know in what form you may get what you want, so keep your options open. Keep them simple and short.

I am eating wholesome, healthy delicious food, in moderation.
I am enjoying success, health, wealth, and happiness.
I am a winner! I am relaxed and peaceful.
I am clearly and confidently expressing myself. I am joyful!
I am loving and nurturing myself and others. I am using everything for my advancement.
I am at peace with myself.
I am enjoying my abundance and prosperity. I am enjoying a loving, supportive, fun relationship. I am relaxed, patient, and paying attention.
My work is interesting, creative, and productive.
I am disciplined and discerning in my work.
I am accepting myself as I am now.
My relationships are filled with laughter and loving. I am clearly and calmly expressing my needs.
I am meeting life's challenges with courage, grace, and acceptance.
I am meeting each moment as an opportunity for growth and learning.
I am accepting other's expression.

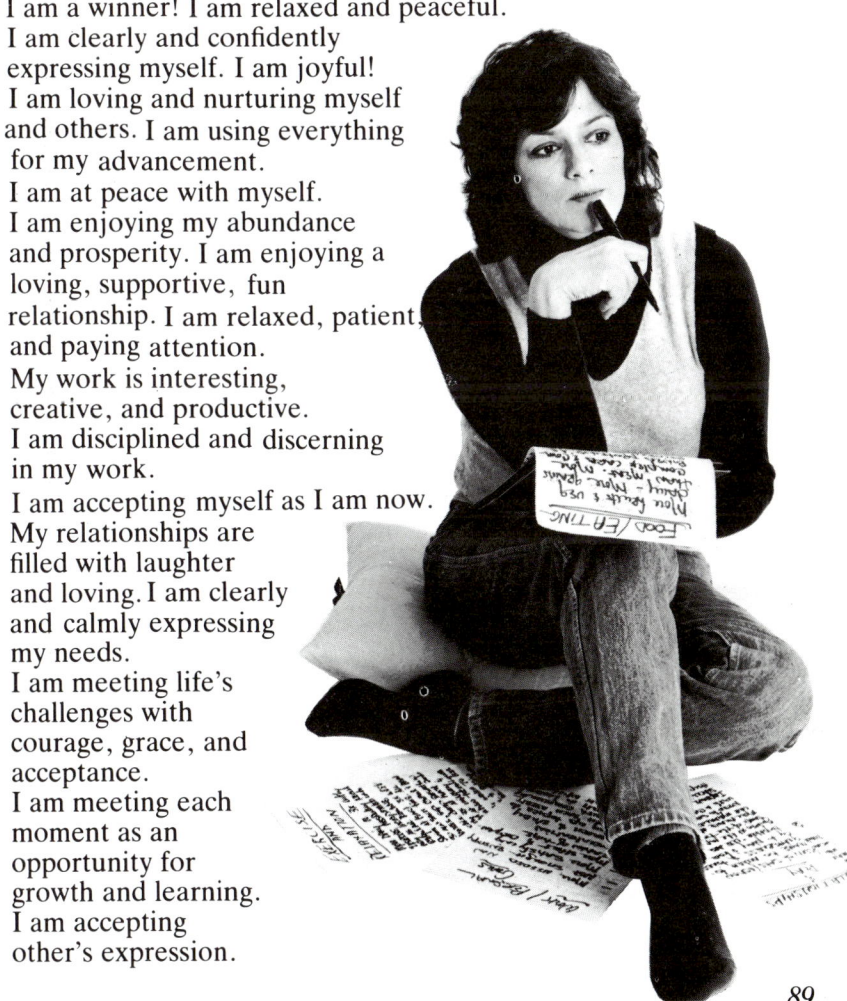

▶ *EXERCISE*

Regular exercise is an important part of your physical, mental, and emotional well-being. The body is similar to an automobile. It usually runs well but it has times when it needs to be repaired. If a car is maintained regularly it runs even better and needs far fewer repairs. Our bodies often keep running for years on end with poor diet and little exercise, but sooner or later it all catches up and there is a breakdown. The body will work better at all times if it gets plenty of maintenance in the form of exercise. Exercise is one of the best treatments for both preventing and managing headaches and other chronic pains.

Exercise makes us look good, and it can also make us feel good. Muscles need exercise or work to stay tuned. Muscles that don't work get flabby and deteriorate. Flabby muscles make it harder for the skeleton to support the body. People often think they feel tired at the end of a day because they have worked too hard, when in reality they have worked their bodies too little.

Exercise increases the heart output, increases the ability of the lungs to inhale and exhale, and increases blood volume, all of which tend to increase overall strength and vitality. Exercise gives a sense of being in touch with, and in control of, the body. People who exercise regularly, even if by just walking briskly every day, tend to be more graceful and confident in their movement.

Exercise can also control overweight, a major factor in low self-esteem. In fact, lack of exercise is more often the cause of overweight than overeating. Gimmicks that promise overnight weight loss are just that — gimmicks. The weight may reduce temporarily, but it inevitably returns. The only way to lose weight and keep it off is through consistent exercise that uses major muscles groups and gets the heart going. Again, simply walking briskly can accomplish those two goals.

Exercise should be thought of as a pleasure, not an obligation or work. There are many, many forms of exercise, so choose one that's just right for you. Do you enjoy exercising indoors with groups on a regular schedule? Try aerobics or dancing classes. Does competition inspire you to action? Try sports such as racquetball and tennis, and team sports such as basketball and volleyball. Do you like to exercise alone or with others? Do you prefer to be indoors or outdoors? Swimming gives the entire body a workout, and is gentle on bones, tendons, and ligaments. Millions of people in the United States have taken up various forms of running and jogging, and bicycling can be both an individual and team sport. Or try horseback riding, hiking, skiing, martial arts, yoga, weight training, rock climbing, sailing, surfing — there are dozens of other possibilities. For city dwellers, a simple walk in the park during a lunch break can change the whole outlook of the day to a positive one.

REGULAR EXERCISE

Regular exercise can help ease or cure the symptoms of headaches, allergies, heart disease, fatigue, tension, and many other illnesses. It tends to equalize the blood flow, cleanse the muscle tissues, equalize the hormonal and chemical balances in the body, boost the immune system by increasing the body's resistance to disease, and cleanse the lungs and increase breathing capacity.

Before beginning any exercise it's a good idea to do some stretching exercises to warm up the body and increase the blood flow to the muscles. This precaution reduces the risk of strains and sprains.

It may help to keep the following pointers in mind when starting out on a new exercise program:

- Be patient with yourself and your body.
- Don't make negative comparisons of yourself to others.
- It takes time to build strength, energy, endurance, coordination, and skill.
- Overdoing may do more harm than good, and can cause injury. It takes time, discipline, and patience to establish a regular exercise routine.
- Chances are excellent that you will be sore during the first couple of weeks of exercise. (This doesn't mean injured, just feeling muscles that haven't been used for a while.) Accept that and keep working through it. After a few weeks the soreness will disappear and your sense of physical fitness and energy will rise steadily. This can be a good time to treat yourself to a massage to relieve and relax sore muscles and to celebrate your new-found fitness.
- Exercising more frequently is more important than how hard you exercise.
- Most specialists recommend exercising for at least thirty minutes at least three days a week.
- Ideally, an exercise routine should be varied enough to improve strength, which is the power of the muscle; flexibility, which is the range of motion in the joints; and endurance, which is cardiovascular fitness or the strengthening of the heart, lungs, and circulatory system.
- If you decide on a formal exercise program, try to choose one that offers training in all three areas.

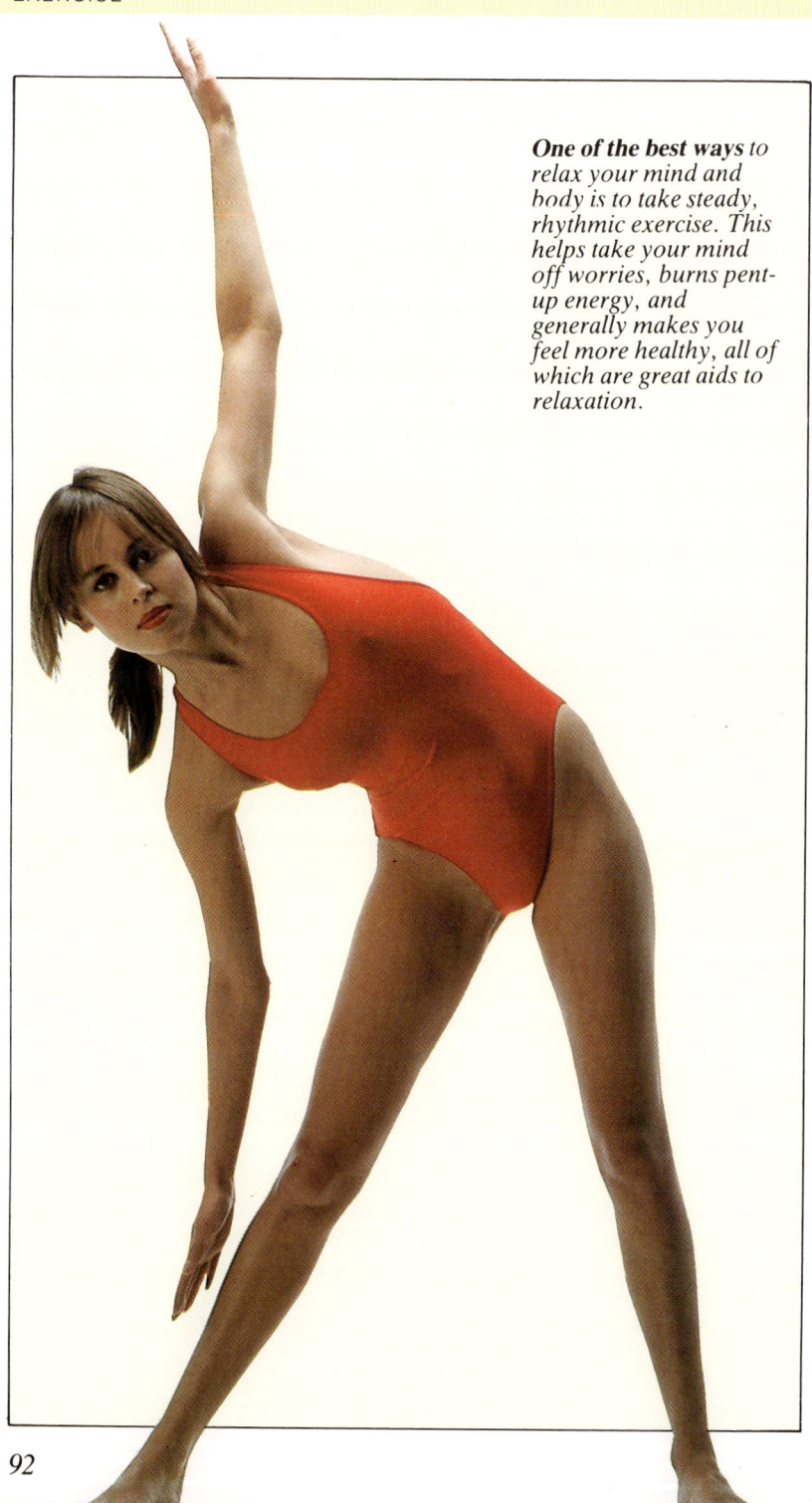

One of the best ways to relax your mind and body is to take steady, rhythmic exercise. This helps take your mind off worries, burns pent-up energy, and generally makes you feel more healthy, all of which are great aids to relaxation.

▶ *RELAXATION*

Relaxation is the opposite of stress. There are many levels of relaxation, from watching television to exercise, to deep relaxation such as sleep, yoga, and meditation. While the lighter levels of relaxation are important, deep relaxation can profoundly affect your ability to cope with stress, change, and the daily demands of life. Deep relaxation helps to discharge tension, both physical and emotional, helps overcome anxiety, promotes peace of mind, and can teach us to listen more sensitively to the messages and needs of our bodies.

Sleep is, of course, a vital form of deep relaxation for which there is no substitute. Deep, relaxed sleep recharges the body by regenerating cells, tissues, and the immune system. Dreaming, or the rapid eye movement (REM) phase of sleep, is an important part of maintaining emotional well-being. Research shows that without dream sleep we may become irritable, restless, or anxious. Sleeping pills suppress dream sleep, so they should be used as infrequently as possible.

Yoga is a practical form of relaxation for the mind and body developed in the Eastern countries. Yoga can bring enhanced strength, flexibility, and grace to the body, and benefits all the organs. Yoga is designed to deeply relax and expand the awareness of the mind and body. It involves specific steps and postures, and breathing exercises.

Massage can be extremely relaxing. It's important to find a well-trained and qualified massage therapist with whom there is a good sense of rapport and trust. Swedish massage is the most common and basic form of healing and relaxing massage. Others include Shiatsu, Neo-Reichian, reflexology, polarity, and Rolfing. Some psychotherapies, including Gestalt, Rogerian, and Hakomi can assist in bringing greater mind *and* body relaxation.

The *Alexander Technique* and the *Feldenkrais Method* are both techniques for re-educating the body into more positive habits and patterns, with a resulting positive change in overall awareness. The Alexander Technique can be especially helpful in relieving chronic back pain. The Feldenkrais Technique focuses on the neuromuscular patterns in the body. It is very gentle and relaxing, whether done in individual sessions or in group sessions called Awareness Through Movement.

Deep-breathing exercises can be done any time or place to reduce stress. When we are stressed we tend to breathe more rapidly and shallowly, or hold our breath. Breathing exercises are usually done in conjunction with yoga and some forms of meditation.

The practice of deep relaxation or *meditation* is an important part of stress management. There are many deep-relaxation techniques. A few are meditation, deep muscle relaxation, self-hypnosis, and biofeedback. What they all have in common is creating an inner state of "passive attention." Passive attention is paying attention without forcing, pushing, or having a goal. Relaxation techniques should be performed without expectations. There is nothing to achieve except getting to know yourself better and coming closer to your center, and that will happen on your own personal timeline. It is a time to be alert without being tense.

Some meditation techniques advocate focusing the mind on a word, a sound, or the breathing. If you suddenly find yourself thinking about work, errands, and so on while meditating, gently bring your attention back to the sound or word. Another technique is to allow the mind to go where it will, and to simply observe it. Watch your thoughts, ideas, and images go by without getting involved. If you do suddenly find yourself involved, gently step back again.

The *"Relaxation Response"* is a combination of Eastern meditative disciplines developed by Harvard professor Herbert Benson. Sit in a quiet place, close your eyes, and silently repeat the word one" over and over for 20 minutes at least twice a day. Concentrating on this single, neutral word focuses the attention away from the demands of everyday life. Benson and others have shown that this technique can help relieve a wide variety of disturbances, including chronic pain, headaches, stomach problems, high blood pressure, and asthma.

In *Progressive Relaxation,* tension is consciously released from the body starting with the toes and slowly working up to the top of the head. It is done by focusing on the part of the body to be relaxed, and then inwardly giving a calm, reassuring instruction to release all tension in the area. Feel every cell, from the marrow of the bones to the skin, relax. Feel the muscles relax and loosen, and go on to the next area. Once an area has been relaxed, don't go back to it.

A variation on this is to take a deep breath, and tighten the muscles of the area to be relaxed. Do not tighten any other muscles except those in the Focus area (this can take some practice). Hold the tightening and the breath as long as possible, and then release both simultaneously with a forceful "whoosh!"

Guided Imagery is a wonderful relaxation method if done without emotional involvement. With this technique you imagine yourself in a profoundly peaceful and relaxing place, usually a beautiful natural setting. There are many narrated cassette tapes with excellent guided imagery meditations on them.

RELAXING EXERCISES

These exercises are designed to help reduce some of the tension in your body and help you relax.

1 Reach up and out with your arms. Stretch all over — yawn if you feel like it. Stretch out and contract the muscles of first one leg and then the other.

2 Raise your arms forward at shoulder height. Let them drop loosely so that they fall past your hips with a "swish." Repeat several times.

3 Stand with your feet slightly apart and your arms raised above your head, the hands nearly touching. Let your arms drop loosely so that they cross in front of you. Raise your arms up again sideways and repeat. Remember to keep your arms relaxed.

Before taking exercise always warm up your muscles with light rhythmic stretching movements. When your muscles feel supple and warm, run on the spot, slowly for one minute then faster for one minute so that you feel slightly out of breath. Then start relaxation exercises that combine exercising all the different muscle groups — legs, arms, neck, chest, back and abdomen — with even, regular deep breathing. The following exercise is a particularly good one for relaxation.

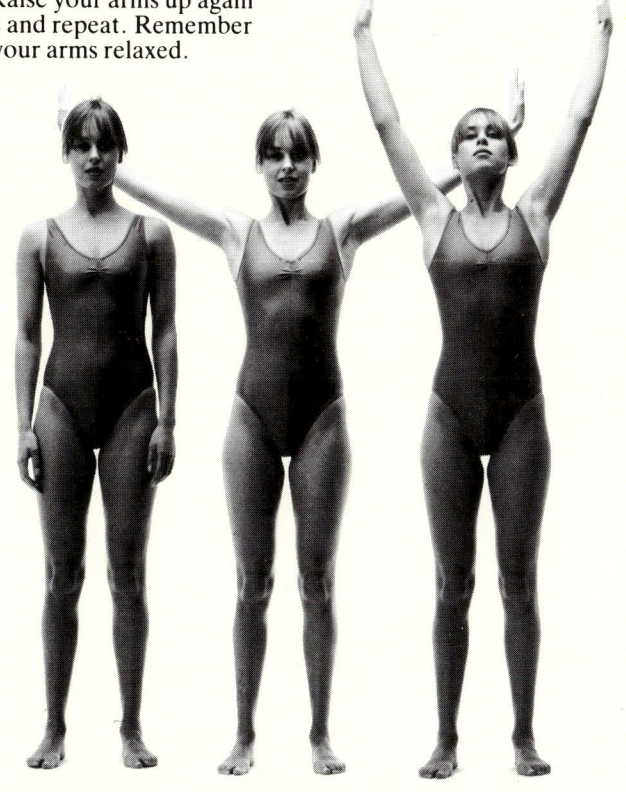